75 Secrets Revealed On Top 15 Diets

The Only Book That Exposes The Pros and Cons of 15 Famous Diets

45 Free Recipes for Breakfast, Lunch & Dinner

Alexis Sanders

--PART 1--

fessionals in the legal, medical, business, accounting, and finance fields.

First Published, 2014

Dedication

To all my readers

About the Author

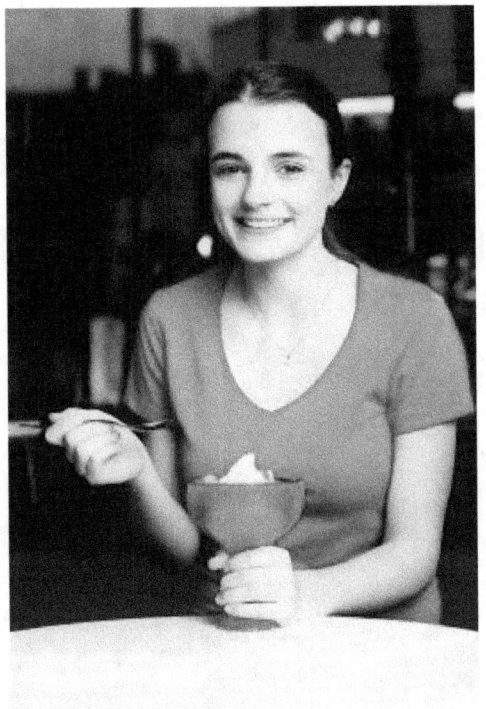

Alexis Sanders is a food photographer. She loves travelling and tasting various cuisines.

It's her first book. She is in the process of writing the 2nd part of this series.

Contact her at: alexis_book@yahoo.com

Table of Contents

INTRODUCTION

Introduction

This is my first book. I hope you will find some valuable information on the Top 15 diets of 2014.

This book is a part of a series of 2 books. This is the 1st part. The 2nd book is on its way. I should be able to publish it within 2-3 months.

Along with each diet, there are 3 recipies in each chapter for breakfast, lunch and dinner.

This book will also help you decide on which diet is most convenient for you. Based on the information provided in this book, you will be able to make a better purchasing decision for your recipe books.

Chapter 1

Secrets about the Anti-Inflammatory Diet

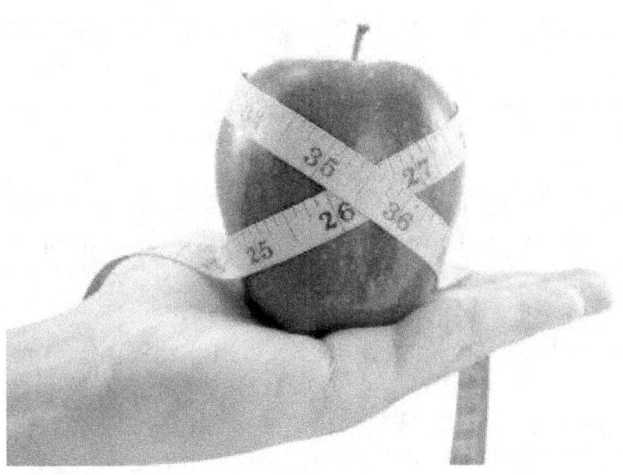

The anti-inflammatory diet, as the name suggests, works with anti-inflammatory food options. Inflammation is the irritation and redness on the surface of the skin.

Generally it occurs as an immunity response towards injury or infection and is beneficial for the body. It is a healing process. But sometimes the itchiness and irritation lingers on for no reason.

This is a harmful situation, because instead of healing, this inflammation can result in decay of tissue, infection or even serious diseases.

The diseases can range from dermatological ailments to tissue and bone decay and even cancer or severe heart disease. This can be prevented by adopting the anti-inflammatory diet.

This diet has been developed by Harvard educated Dr. Weil, who believes that "chronic inflammation can lead to chronic disease".

For this, foods that are healing in nature are adopted in the diet, and inflammatory foods like sugars, oils, and dairy are discarded. Let us look at what you need to know before plunging into this diet.

What it does?

The anti-inflammatory diet is not a diet per se. That is, it is not a program meant primarily for weight loss, though weight loss is still an added benefit. Basically, this diet is meant for removing toxins from the body and healing it.

This is done to realize optimum physical as well as mental well-being which is accomplished by choosing the right food. Unlike most other diets, this diet is not meant for a certain time period.

Its purpose of cleansing the body thoroughly can be accomplished only if it is adopted as a way of life. It also focuses on slowing down the ageing process.

This miraculous diet can help heal as well as prevent various diseases. One can prevent not only skin ailments, but also grave maladies like cancer, rheumatoid arthritis, and heart disease.

How it works?

This works on the principle of satiety of hunger. For this, a lot of fiber is included in the form of fruits, vegetables and whole grains. The recommended daily intake is 2000 to 3000 calories, according to life-style, build and gender. Most of the calories are derived from fats and proteins, and some from carbohydrates.

It is mostly vegetarian but fish is an integral part for the provision of omega-3 fatty acids, and fresh, healing foods are preferred over packaged or processed. Pure water and water-based drinks are recommended for regular and thorough cleansing. It is low sodium and a host of supplements are recommended for vitamins and minerals.

What to avoid?

The anti-inflammatory diet needs you to avoid some food items as well. These are basically the inflammatory foods. You need to take care that you avoid these foods as carefully as you focus on the right foods.

Significant amount of inflammatory consumption will nullify the effect of all the right choices you have made. Alcohol, red meat and dairy products should be avoided as much as possible. Sugars, refined oil and refined grains should also be shown the door. All processed foods, artificial additives, trans fats and saturated fats are a strict no-no for this diet.

Versatile nature

This is one of the most flexible diets as it does not list out meal plans. It only recommends more or less of some foods. No food is black-listed and alcohol is permitted too. It is a 'plan your own meal' kind of diet. But this feature also makes it difficult to stick to.

You may get demotivated after some time. Apart from flexibility in meals, this diet can work perfectly well for vegetarians and vegans. No matter what your preferences are, you just have to mold your choices to suit it. The diet can be made low sodium, gluten free, lactose free and kosher too.

This varied preference makes this diet suitable for one and all. It is good for every age group and can be costly or inexpensive, depending on your choice of ingredients.

Quite well researched

The anti-inflammatory diet may appear to be based on a mere hypothesis. The notion that inflammation can lead to illness and that adopting this diet can reduce inflammation seems theoretical.

But the fact is that this diet can actually help you prevent and cure inflammation-related diseases and age gracefully as well. Though research on this diet has been few and far apart, the results have been astounding. Almost all respondents show signs of improvement in weight control, disease control and overall health.

Still, this diet can be studied more extensively to include various factors and preferences. This will help develop the diet better. In fact, many such studies are under progress. But the difficulty arises because the benefits of this diet can be recorded only after a long period of time.

In any case, there should be no doubt about whether this diet is based on fact or theory.

Working out - the necessary supplement

The diet does not give a plan about working out or physical activity. Yet, Dr. Weil believes that some amount of physical work out should be a part of every diet or every individual's lifestyle.

We all know that working out removes toxins from the body in ways not achievable by any other means. The sweating and perspiration remove harmful agents from the skin, which directly leads to lesser chances of inflammation.

Physical activity cleanses the body thoroughly, reduces stress and acts like icing on the cake for those following this diet. It is entirely up to you to decide the kind and duration of the exercise you would like to do.

So, all in all, the anti-inflammatory diet is a great way of life and can help you achieve the optimum health that one needs and desires. There is no need to think twice.

Give this diet a shot and you will definitely find yourself in a better position in ways beyond weight reduction or health. It will keep your mind active and you will feel better overall.

And the simple key is to ditch bad fats, red meats, excessive amounts of carbohydrates, and instead switch to fresh and wholesome grains, fruits, vegetables and unsaturated fats.

Eating right is the best way to ensure great health.

Now that we know about the diet, let us look at how the actual meals look like. Because the diet is all about choosing the right ingredients and menus, cooking can be quite cumbersome.

You will find a lot of unconventional and never-heard-before recipes and ingredients while on this diet. But nonetheless, they all are delicious and healthy too.

Read on to find three recipes for breakfast, lunch and dinner. All of these recipes are recommended by Dr. Weil himself. You can find more of them on his health site. So, here we go.

RECIPES

Breakfast

The breakfast is recommended to be carbo-hydrate-specific. Cherry quinoa porridge replaces the traditional oatmeal with quinoa. Check out this amazing recipe.

Ingredients

- 1 cup of water
- ½ cup of dried cherries
- 1 tablespoon of honey
- ½ teaspoon of vanilla extract
- ½ cup of dry quinoa
- ¼ teaspoon of powdered cinnamon

Preparation

Combine all ingredients except honey in a pan and heat.
Bring to a boil while stirring constantly. Reduce the heat and let simmer until quinoa is cooked or water evaporates. Top with honey and serve hot. Your delicious breakfast porridge is ready!

Lunch

The lunch should be mildly heavy with enough proteins and fatty acids. Try these awesome roasted chicken rolls for a sumptuous and healthy lunch.

Ingredients
- 2 tablespoons pickle juice
- ¼ teaspoon each of kosher salt and cayenne pepper
- 6 whole wheat or multi-grain flatbreads
- 1 teaspoon of black pepper, cracked
- 1 tablespoon of apple cider vinegar
- ½ cup of low-fat mayonnaise
- 1 roasted chicken, cooled
- 1 ½ cup of red cabbage, chopped

Preparation

Mix pickle juice, mayonnaise and pepper in a bowl and refrigerate. Combine the cabbage, salt, vinegar and cayenne pepper in a bowl and mix thoroughly. Strip the meat off the chicken and cut into small pieces. Add this chicken to mayonnaise and mix well. Take a flatbread and spread the cabbage and chicken mixtures on it evenly. Roll the bread and repeat with the rest of the flatbreads and your yummy lunch rolls are good to go.

Dinner

The ideal anti-inflammatory diet should have at least one fish meal every day. For dinner, you can have this quick and easy recipe of steamed salmon with lemon-scented zucchini.

Ingredients

- 2 small zucchini, finely sliced
- 1 onion, finely sliced
- 1 lemon, finely sliced
- 4 fillets of salmon
- ½ cup of water
- 1 cup of white wine
- ¼ teaspoon each of kosher salt and ground pepper
- Olives (green or black), thinly sliced

Preparation

Take a large Dutch oven and place the onion, lemon, water, wine and zucchini at its bottom. Season the salmon with salt and pepper. Use a greased steamer rack over the mixture and heat until the liquid comes to a boil. Reduce the heat and place the fish on the rack. Cover and steam until the fish is cooked (about 10 minutes). Top the fish

with steaming liquid. Garnish with olives
and serve hot.

Chapter 2

Secrets about the Alkaline Diet

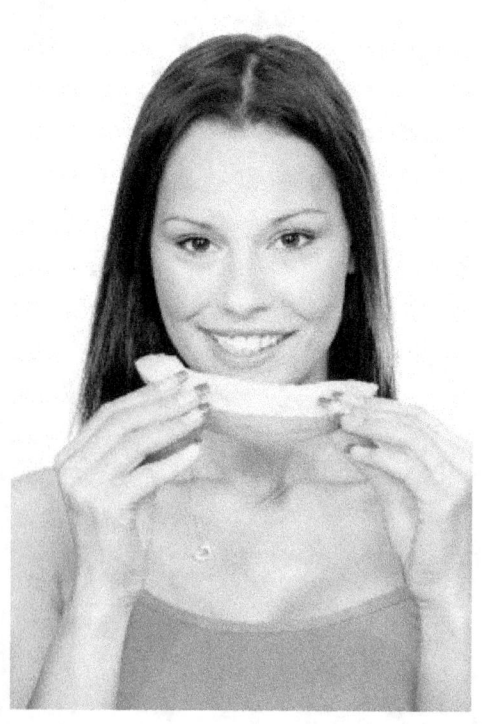

Maintaining a balanced pH level is important. The pH level is used to find out the level of acidity or alkalinity of an object. It is measured from 0-14, with 0 being totally acidic and 14 being totally alkaline. Our body requires a pH level between 7.33 and 7.4. The food that we eat and our hormonal activities discharge an acid or an alkaline base. To find out your pH level, you can test your bodily fluids and find out.

History:

Our ancestors first started out by gathering vegetables, fruits, nuts and other alkaline foods. To counter that, they began hunting and consuming meat and fish. This helped their bodies maintain a balanced acid-alkaline diet, which is very essential for the body. Recently, as agriculture and technology continue to develop, we have swerved from this path, especially with the emergence of fast food and processed food.

Even if we do not get an excess of acidity, our body has alkaline reserves that will help maintain the balance of the body. However, if we consume too many acidic foods, the reserves will not be able to compensate and we will be faced with a lot of health issues. Luckily, the alkaline diet helps us by maintaining the acids in our body and balancing the acid-alkaline ratio.

How it works?

Our lives depend on the balance of our pH levels. If our pH levels cross 7.7 or fall below 7, we will be knocked unconscious and it will lead to a painful death. The diet helps you maintain the pH levels in your body and even help you trim your waist.

The diet mainly focuses on alkaline foods because of our dependence on alkaline-based foods. It promotes the importance of eating fruits, vegetables, nuts, and so on. These foods are rich in calcium and magnesium, among a few that is high on alkaline that help to curb your acid intake.

There are three types of alkaline foods: good, better and best. The best is what we strive for, but we initially start with good. The alkaline diet has been proven by the Dr. Young on its benefits.

Seeing as the diet became popular only recently, there may not be enough statistics and studies. However, many people have come forward and shared their personal experiences on how this diet has changed their lives.

The diet is a long-term process, which means you need to stick to the food you eat.

Benefits:

Our body uses up a lot of energy trying to maintain a balance. If your diet is acidic, it will be harder for your body to compensate, which may lead to depression, exhaustion, anxiety, and so on. Here are a few benefits of this diet that will exonerate these problems:

Balances pH level in blood:

The foods you consume on this diet will help regulate your blood and maintain the recommended pH level.

It is not like your standard diets:

This diet is very different from the usual diets. Our diets consist largely of acid-based foods, which stress the body and reduce your level of immunity, compromising your ability to maintain a healthy body. This does not mean that you should avoid acid-based foods altogether. Maintain your acid intake, but lower the amount you take to meet your body's demands. Make sure your diet consists of about 60-80% of alkaline foods and 20-40% of acidic foods.

Improve your memory and energy levels:

It will take less amount of energy to keep your pH levels in check. Your memory power increases when you are not feeling exhausted.

Easier elimination of waste:

It becomes easier for the body to get rid of waste and cleanse itself. When your cells are healthy, they rid themselves of waste. When your cells are too weak, this opens up the body to infections and diseases.

You look younger:

When your cells are damaged, they cannot perform their functions. If you balance your pH levels, your cells have the ability to heal themselves. This helps in slowing down the process of aging and keeps away diseases.

Tips:

At the time of this writing, there have been no human studies done that prove the benefits of this diet; most of the tests have been conducted in tubes or on animals. It is therefore based on a theory. There is not much coverage on this diet, seeing as it became popular only in 2013. Here are a few tips that can help you with the initial stages of the diet;

- Before you begin your diet, you need to cleanse your body. Go on a cleansing ritual by consuming only liquids for 24 hours.
- Consume 8-9 ounces of tomato juice with a mix of brewer's yeast and wheat germ.
- Drink at least one glass of cranberry juice on a daily basis. Make sure it does not have processed items like sugar in it.
- Make sure you drink a minimum of 8 glasses of water a day. It cleans out the toxins in your body. Add a few drops of lime juice, which is rich in alkaline.
- For the first three days, your intake can consist of only raw foods. When you cook food, the acidity rises.
- 80% of your food intake should include vegetables, fruits, juice, soups, yogurt and brown rice.
- Acid-rich foods can be prepared for less than 20% of your total food intake. On-

ly the bare minimum of meat, coffee, tea, processed foods, sweets, and especially sugar should be consumed.

• Make sure you get enough exercise. It helps increase the level of oxygen in your blood. Excess acid will be removed in many ways, one of which is sweating.

Health benefits:

The alkaline diet has many benefits, including health benefits that will create a better living style. Acid can cause many damages to our body; this diet can help reduce the risk of falling ill with these diseases and prevent them to an extent.

• **Teeth and Gums:** Your mouth becomes acidic when the acid level is high in your body. This causes bacteria and other harmful organisms to grow faster, which may lead to bad breath, mouth ulcers, gum diseases, tooth decay, and so on. After taking up this diet, many people have noted an increase in the strength of their gums and oral health.

• **Immune system:** When your body is healthy, it can digest the nutrients it absorbs. A healthy body will have a better

28

immune system and stronger white blood cells that help fight away diseases. Infectious bacteria or virus will stand a better chance of being defeated when your immune system is healthy.

• **Pain:** Excess acid is controlled by magnesium, which is an essential nutrient for the body. The greater the amount of magnesium used, the more your body feels pain. Following this diet will help you increase your magnesium levels. It will destroy acid deposits and reduce pain and inflammation.

• **Weight loss:** This diet helps in healthy weight loss. Anyone can follow this diet and slim down and tone their body. At the same time, their metabolism also increases.

• **Decreases risk of acidosis and alkalosis:** When the pH level falls below 7.3, it is known as acidosis. The exact opposite is alkalosis. These are diseases that impact a person physically and mentally. This diet helps curb both diseases.

RECIPES

Breakfast
Spelt porridge

Ingredients
- 1 cup water
- 1/3 thin powdered spelt
- Agave syrup
- ¼ tablespoon of vanilla (no alcohol)
- 2-3 tablespoons of cherries
- Assortment of nuts, berries, and milk

Preparation
Take a bowl and pour 1 cup of water into it. Add the spelt, syrup, vanilla, cherries and nuts and berries and mix them. Heat mixture on a stove at medium heat, and once cooked, put into a bowl. Top with fruits of your choice, and pour milk over the ingredients. Your breakfast is ready! If you want to add more nuts or milk, feel free to do so.

Lunch
Grilled Vegetable Pesto Pasta

Ingredients
- 1 cup basil leaves

- 3 tablespoons hemp hearts (preferably raw)
- ¼ cup of cashews
- ¼ cup of olive oil
- 1 clove garlic, minced
- Sea salt
- 1 packet brown penne noodles
- 1 tablespoon pinched sea salt
- 4-5 capsicum
- 2 onions, chopped
- 3 zucchini, sliced
- 4 carrots, chopped
- 1-2 eggplant (small), diced
- 1 asparagus
- 3 tablespoons olive oil (virgin)
- 2 tablespoons pinched sea salt
- Cherry tomatoes, diced

Preparation
Place the first six ingredients into a blender. Blend until mixture becomes a paste. Set aside. Cook pasta according to the instructions on the package. Pour in the pesto sauce. Next, take your vegetables and toss them with salt and olive oil. Grill the vegetables on a grill until they are slightly charred. Place the vegetables with the pesto pasta and mix. Season with the salt and use pepper if you want. Taste and garnish ac-

cordingly. You can serve this with fresh salad to make it more filling. To make the salad, take cabbage, carrots, zucchini, and cherry tomatoes (for the added flavour). You can be creative and add your own ingredients. Toss and add a little bit of sea salt and olive oil.

Dinner
Cosy Raw Vegetable soup with peas, carrots, ginger and cilantro

Ingredients
- 2 cups of roughly chopped carrots

- ½ cup fresh peas

- 1 tablespoon sliced shallot

- ½ piece of cut ginger

- 1/8 cup of lime juice

- 2 cups of water

- ½ avocado

- ½ teaspoon sea salt

- Hazelnut oil

- Cut cilantro

Preparation

Place all the ingredients into a blender. Slowly blend the ingredients until they are roughly chopped and then increase the blender to high for 3-4 minutes. Open the blender to see if there is steam. Taste and add seasoning accordingly. Pour into bowls and add hazelnut oil and lots of cilantro for the added taste. You can serve it with slices of bread. Because this is raw, it retains its flavour and its nutrients. Add more vegetables if you want to.

Chapter 3

Secrets about the Mediterranean Diet

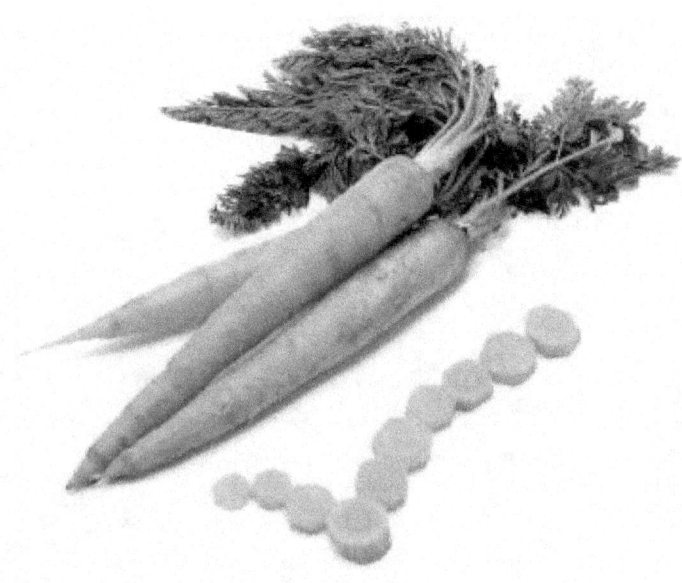

Do you want to lose weight? Follow a healthy diet? Give up on processed food?

There is a way! This diet is based on the way of life of the people in the Mediterranean region, who lead a healthier lifestyle than their European counterparts. Interested in the Mediterranean diet? You will be happy to know that it is healthy and tasty!

Of course, when we think of Mediterranean food, we probably imagine pasta or a nice tasty pizza. Yes, these foods are a part of the Mediterranean culture, but when we talk about a balanced diet, they do not match our needs. The traditional diet consists mainly of vegetables, olive oil, fruits, nuts, legumes, and fish.

Nutrients:

The diet consists of a variety of healthy fats that actually has been proved to help you lose weight! Olive oil, one of the main ingredients used in the diet, is rich in mono-unsaturated fats and helps in reducing lipo-protein. Several nuts and canola oil include linolenic acid, which is a type of omega-3 acid and important for our sustenance. Fish like sardines, tuna, and salmon, are rich in omega-3 fatty acids.

Some important nutrients are found in this diet:

Calcium: It is vital for maintaining bone density, and people, especially women, need to get a lot of calcium. Make sure you consume at least 1,000-1,300 milligrams per day. Eating yogurt, cereals and milk will help.

Fiber: An adult should get a daily dosage of 22-34 grams to encourage proper digestion. Following a Mediterranean diet will help you get the required amount.

Vitamins: Vitamins are one of the most essential nutrients necessary for any being, especially Vitamin B-12 and Vitamin D. Adults should get a recommended daily dosage of 2.4 mg and 15 mg respectively. Yogurt, dairy, and cereals will help you reach your goal.

Potassium: This is another important nutrient necessary for our sustenance. The recommended daily dosage for an adult is 4,700 milligrams. Eating fruits and vegetables will help you maintain your potassium levels. Banana is especially rich in potassium.

The Mediterranean diet became well known in the 90s. Even though there were many studies undertaken, it spread to other parts of the world in the 90s. Most people considered this diet to be a bit of a puzzle. The fat consumption in these regions was quite high, yet the people were healthy. In fact, they were less prone to heart disease, cancer, diabetes and many other diseases. According to a study conducted by Harvard, the life expectancy of a person can increase too! This is one of many secrets of this nourishing diet.

It is important for us to understand that a good, healthy meal goes a long way for us in the future. When you prepare a Mediterranean meal, include an array of choices. This will help our body get the highest intake of vitamins, minerals and other important nutrients. Another increasing health problem is high blood pressure, often caused by the excessive consumption of sodium. To prevent high blood pressure and reduce it, we can use herbs as a substitute for salt. This will also enhance the flavors of the dishes.

Before we move further, we need to know what foods are mainly consumed on the Mediterranean diet:

- Every meal must include vegetables, fruits, nuts, olive oil, spices, legumes, and whole grains.
- Fish can be consumed on a weekly basis.
- Poultry products like chicken can be consumed on a weekly basis or twice a week.
- Red meat is fattening and can lead to many health issues if consumed excessively. Limit it to once a month.
- Water is essential, especially for this diet. Make sure you drink at least six glasses of water a day.

Primary benefits:

The Mediterranean diet was formulated for more than just weight loss; in fact, it focuses more on the health aspect rather than weight loss, unlike most other diets.

There are three main reasons you would want to follow this diet: to improve your health, prevent diseases and to lose weight. We should understand that eating healthy food is not the only thing necessary to maintain a balanced diet. Physical exercise is also important to maintain your body weight and lead a healthy life. The Mediterranean diet stresses this; an active lifestyle coupled with healthy food leads to a healthy life.

A diet will not work if you overindulge. We need to eat properly proportioned meals and drink a lot of water. Water is especially important to rid the body of its toxins. The Mediterranean diet emphasizes on the importance of consuming water. Another important liquid that is a part of the diet is wine. A glass of red wine a day makes you less susceptible to heart disease.

There is no single diet that you can follow. The Italian diet is not the same as the French; their diet is not the same as the Greek. Choose which diet you would like to follow according to your convenience.

If you want to change your diet, but you are intimidated by the Mediterranean diet, here are a few points to change your mind:

• Follow the traditional style of the Mediterranean diet. The present Mediterranean scenario has become infused with Western ideas. Fast foods have become popular in European countries.

• This diet is cheap; you do not have to worry about excessive expenditure. The ingredients are simple and can be bought at your local grocery store.

39

• Many studies have proved this diet can prevent many diseases like cancer, blood pressure and so on.

• It is tasty and healthy. Do not over-indulge, but rather, eat small portions every few hours. Wait for an hour, and if you are hungry, eat a fruit or a bowl of vegetables.

Added benefits:

The closer you get to the perfect, traditional Mediterranean diet, the healthier you become. The possibility of contracting diseases decreases etc.

How do you know if you have prepared proper portions? Here are a few tips to ensure your servings do not exceed the prescribed daily amount.

• Meat: 60-70 grams
• Dairy: Eat at least one cup of yogurt and not more than 25-30 grams of cheese.
• Vegetables: Eat a lot of green, leafy vegetables. Other vegetables are also important for your body; eat at least half a bowl.
• Fruits: Eat a bowl of mixed fruits like grapes, oranges, watermelon and so on, as they are rich in minerals and vitamins.

- Whole wheat grains: Substitute white rice with brown rice. It is tastier and healthier. You can eat pasta too, with bread.
- Nuts: Eat at least a few almonds or groundnuts a day. They are good for your blood and prevent diseases.
- Wine: Make sure you do not consume too much wine. Stick to red wine and limit the amount to one glass (if you are female) or two glasses (if you are male).
- Legumes: Beans are good for your health; eat at least a bowl of beans.
- Physical exercise: Exercise a lot. It is as important as a balanced diet. It will keep you fit and healthy.

Eating a healthy diet is important for people of all age groups, especially middle-aged persons. When you adopt one of the healthiest diets, it transports you to a place of cultural diversity. The Mediterranean consists of 16 countries surrounding the sea. Each of these places is unique and filled with beauty. Traditionally, people from the Mediterranean would work for their meal. The labor to get the fresh ingredients and eating a balanced diet kept the older generation healthy and fit.

Interesting facts:

• This diet focuses only on food: This is a myth, as food is just one part of the diet. Physical exercise and portioning are also integral to living a healthy life

• Prevents Spina Bifida: Spina Bifida is a birth defect that causes incomplete growth of the spine. The Mediterranean diet helps prevent this defect.

• Less is more: This does not apply to the traditional diet; in fact, studies show that you must eat until you are full to be healthy.

What goes where:

Since the diet mainly consists of fruits and vegetables, here is a list of them:

• Yellow and red peppers, carrots and radishes are rich in potassium and Vitamin C. They go well with almost all dishes from the diet. Tomatoes, squash, and beets are also an important part of your diet and contain many essential nutrients.

• Green, leafy vegetables are abundant in vitamins and fiber. Broccoli, peas, and beans are among those that are especially favored in the Mediterranean diet. Try making a bowl of just green vegetable salad with a few drops of olive oil and lemon juice for taste.

• Eggplant is one of the most recurring vegetables in the diet. You can add it to anything from noodles to lasagna or grill the eggplant and be creative with the toppings. Cauliflower is also another vegetable that is seen in many dishes. Its abundant nutrients makes it a popular vegetable.

RECIPES

Breakfast
Mediterranean Egg Muffins

For a healthy and filling breakfast, here's a wonderful recipe for egg muffins. You can refrigerate these muffins and keep them up to seven days!

Ingredients
- 1 tablespoon of olive oil
- Dozen eggs
- 2 cups of spinach, finely chopped
- ¾ cup of tomatoes, finely chopped
- 1 teaspoon of garlic powder
- ¼ cup of cheese, crumbled
- ½ tablespoon of salt
- ¼ tablespoon pepper

Preparation
Heat a pan over medium heat. Pour some olive oil into the pan so that the vegetables do not stick. In the meantime, pre-heat your oven at 370 degrees. Put the spinach and tomatoes into the pan and cook them until the spinach turns a bright green. Add the eggs to the vegetables, along with the crumbled cheese, salt and pepper. Mix well and

heat for 2-3 minutes. Take a tin muffin tray and fill ¾ of the cups. This allows the muffins to rise. Put it in the oven for 18-22 minutes. Your breakfast is ready!

Lunch
Mediterranean Quinoa Salad

Ingredients
- 3 cups of quinoa, cooked
- 3 tablespoons of capers
- 3 tablespoons of nuts (preferably pine)
- 2-3 spoons of spring onion, finely chopped
- 2-3 spoons of herbs (preferably dill)
- 2-3 spoons of garlic, minced
- 1-2 spoons of lemon juice
- ¼ cup olive oil
- Seasoning

Preparation
Put the quinoa in a big bowl. Add all the ingredients in the same order as given above. Add salt and pepper in the end for seasoning. Mix well. Lunch is ready! Include grapes and cherry tomatoes on the side for a complete lunch.

Dinner
Savory Dinner Crepes

Ingredients

- 3 eggs
- ½ cup water
- 1 cup whole wheat flour
- ¼ cup flax seeds
- ¼ spoon salt
- ¼ cup parsley
- Feta cheese
- Chopped roasted peppers
- Green olives
- Olive oil
- Salmon

Preparation

Take three eggs and crack them into a blender, making sure no egg shells fall in. Pour ½ cup of water into the blender. Add 1 cup of white whole wheat flour to the mixture. Add salt and olive oil, and garlic if you want (make sure the garlic is roasted to give it a nice flavor, and do not add more than 1-2 cloves). Add ¼ cup of parsley or any other herb you want. Blend the ingredients. Meanwhile, leave a pan on the stove over medium heat. Pour the mixture into the pan. Tilt the pan to make sure the crepe fills the pan. Wait for a minute or two and then flip the crepe over. Take the crepe and place it on a plate. If you are making more than one, make sure you place parchment paper between the crepes to avoid sticking. Put the cheese, peppers, green olives and any other ingredient of your choice. Here we are using salmon. Place all these ingredients in the crepe and roll it. Your dinner is ready!

Chapter 4

Secrets about the Flexitarian Diet

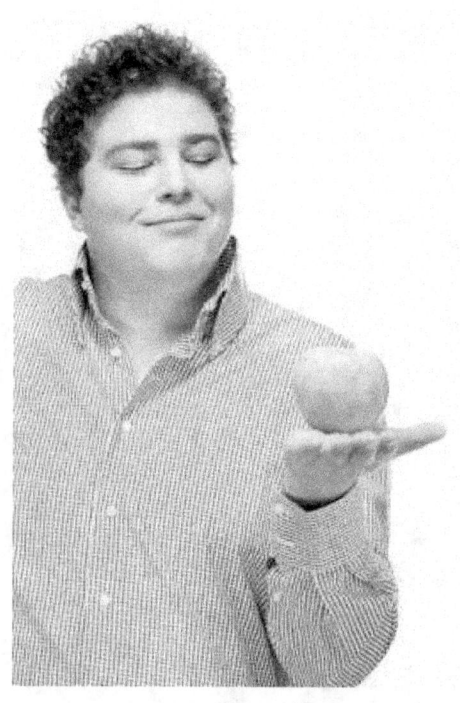

If you are healthy, you have everything. Who thought that the key to a carefree life would lie in our everyday diet plan? Many people take health for granted; but a well-balanced, nutritious diet is all it takes to get rid of the health issues that we face. This is where the much recommended Flexitarian Diet comes into picture.

The word 'flexitarian' is an amalgamation of the words flexible and vegetarian. It requires a person to eat mostly vegetarian food, occasionally indulging in meat.

It is one of the most popular and beneficial diets among both dieticians and the public. Dawn Jackson Blatner, a well-known author and dietician, is the creator of this semi-vegetarian diet.

Her book, 'The Flexitarian Diet' is an encyclopedia of all things flexitarian, containing recipes, guides and general information about this famous diet. Here are the secrets of the Flexitarian Diet that will amaze you and make it irresistible:

Claims and Benefits

Dawn Jackson Blatner claims that her creation lowers heart disease, diabetes and cancer. According to Blatner, her diet can increase a flexitarian's lifespan by up to 3.6 years ! Moreover, it improves your immunity, thereby increasing your energy. All you have to do is be flexitarian. Apart from its proud claims, there are many benefits to this diet. The primary ones are as follows:

- It decreases the daily allowance of your calorie intake, thereby increasing your stamina. The fruits, vegetables and grains taken as substitutes for meats keep you light and active.
- It lowers your cholesterol and keeps heart disease at bay. As a result, a flexitarian leads a healthier life when compared to other meat eaters.
- It does not result in any side effects, as there is least consumption of packaged foods and preservatives. As the food is homemade, hygiene is maintained.
- The diet is abundant in fiber, nutrients and vitamins.
- It decreases the regular intake of saturated fat by 15%.
- The 'calorie deficit' helps in reducing one's weight.
- The wholesome eating leads to a steady weight loss.

- It is the most vegetarian way to lose weight.
- It adds years to your life.
- It lowers your blood pressure and stabilizes sugar levels.
- It increases your protein intake to a great extent.

How It Works

The Flexitarian Diet consists of mainly five food groups: fruits and vegetables, sugar and spice, new meat, dairy and whole grains.

While the rest are self-explanatory, 'new meat' refers to swaps such as eggs, nuts, tofu and lentils. It provides a five-week diet plan consisting of breakfast, lunch and dinner.

Flexitarians can either swap recipes or follow the general diet plan. The calorie intake for each meal is as follows:

- **Breakfast**-300
- **Lunch**-400
- **Dinner**-500

The above given intake is a typical Flexitarian Diet. However, it can be modified to accommodate more calories depending on height, weight, and gender. Hence, this diet is flexible, as it does not restrict a dieter to a limited number of calories. In fact, it compromises according to your needs, provided that the food groups are consumed.

Fruits and Vegetables

They are an important part of the diet – oranges, spinach, apples, corn, lentils, radish, and so on. They balance the nutrient and vitamin levels.

Additional Benefits

Apart from the primary benefits, there are a few other advantages to this popular diet:

- You could lose up to 30 pounds, provided the diet is followed for 6 to 12 months! As a flexitarian can eat meat occasionally, there is no sacrifice of taste.

- Research proclaims that this diet leads to a healthy weight and consumption of fresh and seasonal fruits.
- It makes you more eco-friendly! Studies tell us that by eating less meat, we help in reducing the greenhouse emissions to some extent.
- This diet includes gluten-free meals.
- This diet helps in saving money as fruits, vegetables, tofu, and nuts are less costly than meat and poultry.
- As its name suggests, the diet is flexible and offers various options.
- The diet encourages you to make one change per day. There is no need to hurry; you can take one step at a time.
- It maintains variety, moderation and balance in foods and the body.
- It is a good option for vegetarians opting for a healthy balance of both veg and non-veg.
- It encourages you to be creative with meal planning.

Tips to Swap

It is a common problem for those on strict diets to completely renounce their 'meat life'. However, the Flexitarian Diet does not force its takers to sacrifice a lot.

This diet suggests the principle of swapping. Meats and other foods are swapped with healthier alternatives like tofu, lentils, nuts, tuna, peas, and beans. These healthier options are called 'new meats'.

The diet has a clever aspect to it as it aims at reducing the calories while still retaining taste. Here are a few tips to swap your unhealthy cravings with delicious, healthy ones:

- Swap the sour cream on your taco salad with the finger-licking goodness of guacamole.
- Put away the dreaded shredded cheese on your pizza for a pine nut-topped flat bread.
- Swap the spicy turkey chili with a healthier alternative, vegetarian chili.
- Swap chicken breast for a delicious tofu cutlet.

- Do away with the meat sauce for your pasta. Make it healthier by adding white beans and fresh basil instead.
- Swap your regular lunch meat sandwich with lentil salad in a whole grain pita.
- Get rid of that cheesy, fattening hamburger for a juicy black bean burger instead.
- Swap the high-cholesterol shrimp stir fry for an edamame stir fry.
- Opt for a vegetarian refried bean burrito instead of a steak one.

Undoubtedly, the Flexitarian Diet is the best one you can come across. With so many foods to choose from, one cannot say no. It makes you healthy, without requiring you to give up meat. With such a promising diet plan, you don't think twice before you eat.

You don't starve, so you won't be compelled to binge on your 'cheat days' either.

In a world filled with junk food, it often requires extra focus to stay on a diet, which is all the more reason to find one that will not only make us healthy, but also satisfies our taste buds.

Heather Morgan once said that, "Every time you eat or drink something, you are either feeding disease or fighting it".

Now we have to decide whether we want to feed or fight our diseases. Every time we have a meal, we need to keep this in mind. The Flexitarian Diet gives you so much more than just healthy food.

So why not start today and live this promise? Eat healthy, stay healthy.

RECIPES

We just don't want to leave you in the exciting world of a flexitarian diet, clueless about what dishes to eat to remain steadfast. There are many recipes you can try to fill your tummies with tasty food. We recommend to you some of the best, easy-to-prepare dishes that will keep you both healthy as well as happy!

Breakfast
Apple and Almond Butter Toast

Ingredients
- 1 slice of whole wheat bread
- 1 ½ tablespoon of almond butter or peanut butter
- 1 slice of apple

Preparation
Toast the bread and spread almond or peanut butter on it. Accompany the toast with a slice of apple. This breakfast will give you a great start for the day.

Lunch
Brown Rice with Edamame Stir Fry

Ingredients

- 1 cup of hot cooked brown rice
- 1 red bell pepper, sliced
- 1 clove garlic, minced
- ¼ cup of 100% pineapple juice
- 2 teaspoons of sesame oil
- ½-inch chunk of fresh gingerroot, peeled and grated
- ¾ cup of fresh edamame beans
- Pinch of crushed red pepper flakes
- Dash of salt

Preparation: Sauté the garlic, red bell pepper,, salt, and ginger in oil over medium heat for three minutes. A striking feature of this recipe is that lean steak strips are swapped with the edamame. Once you are done with the sauté, you can add the pineapple juice and fresh edamame beans. Cook for about eight minutes over high heat. Add the cooked brown rice and enjoy this delicious meal! This dish serves one flexitarian.

Dinner
Cilantro-Lime Pesto with Orzo

Ingredients

- 1 clove garlic, minced

- 1 teaspoon of olive oil
- 1 cup of fresh cilantro
- 2 ounces of cooked tuna or salmon
- 1 tablespoon of pine nuts
- 1 teaspoon of olive oil
- ¼ cup of roasted red peppers (in a water packed jar), chopped and drained
- ¼ cup of corn kernels
- ¼ cup (2 ounces) of uncooked whole grain orzo (rice-shaped pasta)

Preparation

Dinner is always the risky meal in a diet. It has to be light, extremely healthy and full of energy. Most importantly, dinner should be had as early as possible.

Keeping these points in mind, this diet swaps black beans with tuna, salmon or any other fish. It is simple to prepare this dish. Cook orzo as per the instructions mentioned on the package. Make a puree of garlic, pine nuts, lime juice, cilantro and oil in a food processor or a blender to make the pesto. Once the pesto is done, you can cook it with the orzo and the rest of the ingredients. There, you just prepared a delicious, yet light flexitarian dinner for yourself!

Chapter 5

Secrets about the Weight Watchers Diet

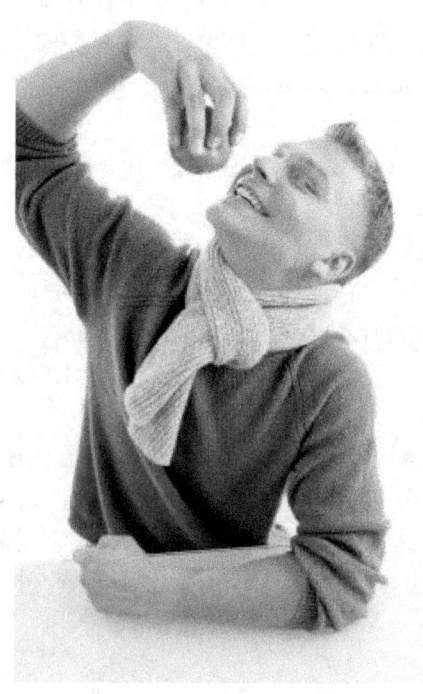

You are what you eat. Be it the delicious pasta you hogged last night or the oatmeal you just had this morning, every meal that we gorge on has an impact on our body that can be good or bad. To maintain a good balance of this impact, we must have a proper diet. Often, diets restrict the intake of our favorite foods, making us unsatisfied.

Although we somehow accept this limitation, we tend to slip whenever we see a tasty meal lying temptingly in front of us. We often assume that diets are meant to be restrictive, but the Weight Watchers Diet is an exception. Rather than restricting any type of food, this diet allows the consumption of all kinds of food. It is nothing like the usual diets, where one has to starve until they lose some weight.

Instead, this diet assigns points to proportions of fats, fiber, carbohydrates and protein in a dish. The people who undertake this diet become members of the Weight Watchers program. They form an integral part of the group. Here are the secrets of this popular diet that demand your undue attention:

Claims and Benefits: This diet improves the eating habits of people and their lifestyles. It also claims that those undertaking this diet lose twice as much weight as those on a standard weight loss program for 12 months.

The primary benefits of the Weight Watchers Diet are as follows:

• There is no need to reduce or alter the intake of any food items. The diet allows all kinds of dishes.
• Weight Watchers is not a diet at all. It allows the consumption of all foods in specific proportions.
• It leads to gradual weight loss with no health hazards.
• The diet is very balanced and has no deficiency of any kind.
• It is a customized weight loss program and caters to every individual's personal needs and requirements.
• The members are regularly updated about the latest nutrition and exercise-related information.
• People get to know each other better through this program. This strengthens the community aspect and boosts motivation.

How it Works

To follow the diet, you have to register as a member first. The main principle of this diet is the Plus Points Target. The dieters are allowed to eat all kinds of foods.

There are no restrictions placed on the types of dishes consumed. There is only one condition – the different foods need to be consumed in specific proportions. This helps in reducing weight without restricting one's appetite.

Once you become a member, you can easily find the point values of about 40,000 types of foods on the website of Weight Watchers. Processed foods have high points, so one must consume them in small quantities, whereas fruits and vegetables carry zero points.

This means one can have as many fruits and vegetables as he/she likes. The main categories under this diet are proteins, carbohydrates, fiber and fats.

Weight Watchers also conducts regular meetings where members can share their success stories and discuss other weight loss-related tips with each other.

Facts

Apart from its key benefits, there are lots of things a regular dieter may not know about the Weight Watchers Diet. Perhaps after reading these interesting facts, you would want to join the Weight Watchers club too. Here they are:

• You can choose any weight loss program available online of your choice. The diet does not require you to follow one diet plan. It has a wide variety to choose from depending on one's gender, age, weight, and so on.

• You are bound to lose three times more weight if you attend weekly meetings. Who thought slimming would be this easy?

• If you are not successful in following the diet, or the plan you have chosen is not working out for you, there is no need to worry.

The Weight Watchers get-togethers are the solution for all your worries. This is the place where members share their recipes and weight loss tips with each other. Who knows, maybe you can find the weight loss tip you've been yearning for in one such gathering.

•   If you are unable to attend the meetings, you can easily access the weight loss programs online.
•   If the diet is followed strictly, you can lose up to 2 pounds per week!

Tips:
- As a beginner, it is hard to keep track of all the do's and don'ts. It becomes hard to follow the diet. We have to maintain a balance between work, house chores, mind and body. They have a huge impact on our health. We need the right course of action to follow this diet properly. Here are a few health tips that will help you to keep this balance intact:
- Exercise regularly.
- Make alterations in your diet and eat everything in specific quantities.
- Water is the key to healthy living. Hydrate yourself with 1.5 to 2 liters of water every day.
- Reduce your fat intake.
- Munch on your favorite fruits and veggies five times a day.

Ingredients to Avoid

Even though this diet allows all kinds of food, some people may go overboard with this freedom, eating too much and ruining their diets. Keep in mind to not have too much of these: flour breads, fruit-flavored yogurt, and breakfast cereal. Be aware of the proportions you consume. Too much of a good thing is bad.

This might be the first time you have come across a diet that permits you to eat anything and everything. After reading about all its claims and benefits, one is bound to be a Weight Watcher – a diet that is healthy and fun at the same time.

How often do you come across a diet plan like this one?

RECIPES

As mentioned earlier, the Weight Watchers Diet has no limitations. It is only concerned with the quantity of intake of fibers, proteins, carbohydrates and fats. Keeping this in mind, we recommend to you the tastiest Weight Watchers recipes you will come across:

Breakfast Sandwich

Ingredients
- 1 English muffin
- 3 eggs, scrambled
- Onion rings
- 1 strip of turkey bacon

Preparation:
Toast a high-fiber, light muffin and top with the remaining ingredients. This meal is a rich source of carbohydrates, protein and fiber.

Lunch

Chiles and Basil with Thai-Style Ground Turkey

Ingredients

- Regular rice or coconut rice
- 3 garlic cloves, finely chopped
- 1 pound of ground turkey
- 1 jalapeno, seeded and finely chopped
- 1 tablespoon of Asian fish sauce (nam pla)
- 1 tablespoon of peanut oil
- Lime wedges
- ½ teaspoon of sugar
- 1 tablespoon of ginger root, finely chopped
- 1 fat scallion (white and light green parts only)
- ½ cup of fresh regular or Thai basil, chopped
- 1 tablespoon of soy sauce
- ¼ teaspoon of finely grated lime zest

Preparation

Whisk sugar, lime juice, lime zest, soy sauce and fish sauce in a small bowl. If the fish sauce is too salty, add only two teaspoons. You can add more if the dish requires it. Over medium to high heat, heat oil in a large dish. Add chopped scallion, ginger, garlic and jalapeno. Keep cooking the ingredients for a minute until they are slightly softened, then add the turkey. Cook the meat for 5 to 7 minutes until it is no longer pink.

Stir in the soy sauce mixture. Cook the dish for a minute, until the flavors rise. After the meal is cooked, remove the pan from the dish. Add some basil and sliced green scallions. Your dish is ready! You can serve it with regular rice or coconut rice. Add some lime wedges for garnishing. Indulge yourself in a tasty, yet nutritious lunch. This dish serves four.

Dinner
Veggie Wontons
Ingredients
- 20 Wonton papers
- ¼ cup of uncooked napa cabbage, shredded
- 1 large egg, beaten
- ¼ cup of fresh shiitake mushrooms, chopped
- 1 tablespoon of fresh ginger root, minced
- 1 tablespoon of fresh cilantro, minced
- ½ teaspoon kosher salt
- 1 tablespoon garlic, minced
- 3 tablespoons of canned water chestnuts, drained and chopped
- 1 tablespoon of hoisin sauce
- 1 tablespoon of low-sodium soy sauce

- Cooking spray
- ½ cup of firm tofu, well drained and crumbled
- 2 medium scallions, chopped
- ¼ cup of carrots, shredded

Preparation

Line two baking sheets with cooking spray and parchment paper. Preheat the oven to 375 degrees Fahrenheit.
Take cilantro, mushrooms, carrot, garlic, ginger, salt, egg, and tofu in a large bowl.

Add scallions, soy sauce, hoisin sauce, cabbage and water chestnuts and stir well. Fill each wonton paper with one and a half teaspoons of the mixture in the center.

Now wet two adjacent wonton edges with your fingertip using water. To make a triangle, fold the wrapper over the filling and press the edges lightly.

Place the wontons on the baking sheets and spray them with cooking spray. Bake the wontons for 10 to 15 minutes until they turn light brown.

Chapter 6

Secrets about the Biggest Loser Diet

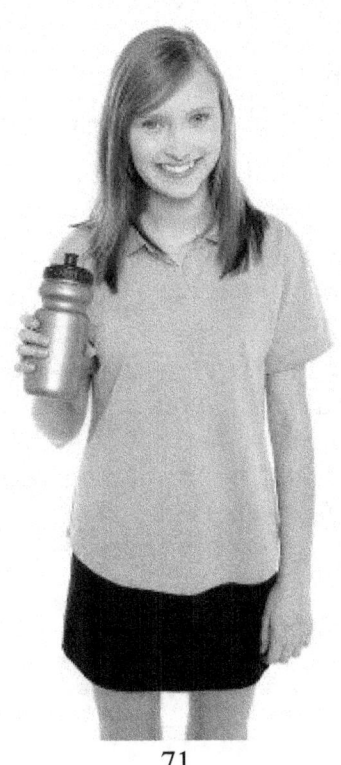

Have you ever watched NBC's *The Biggest Loser*? It is a popular show that focuses on reducing weight by balancing meals and physical exercise. The show became famous for its numerous diets and 100% satisfaction.

The show was started in America because of its growing levels of obesity, but it is broadcasted in close to 90 countries! It became popular because of its methods, and Australia now has their own show.

You can make your own plan at home to help you strengthen your body and mind, lose weight and decrease your blood pressure.

The diet entails a lot of hard work and dedication. It is also a bit expensive, which is why specialists feel people might not see a permanent effect. If you are interested in following this diet, you need to pick one of the "Biggest Loser books" that you can adhere to. This is important, so make sure you choose a cookbook that you are comfortable with.

How it works:

The diet helps you lose weight by eating nutritious food and exercising. If you have a diet plan, make sure you stick to it. Every day you have to write in your food journal. This helps you know how much you have eaten and your eating capacity.

The food you eat should be rich in proteins, calcium, good fats like omega-3, and carbohydrates. The diet gives you the best fiber intake, which is essential for weight loss.

It is important to construct your diet according to your level of obesity and health problems. Make sure your diet helps you in the best way it can.

Prepare yourself to work hard and change your eating patterns. The diet needs absolute commitment and works only on a long-term basis. Stop in between; you will gain back all the weight you lost.

Make sure you control your intake of fatty foods, because they can damage your health and cause health issues, like high cholesterol and blood pressure.

Benefits:

The Biggest Loser diet has many benefits that has made it so appealing to the masses.

It largely concentrates on reducing your intake of calories. This has helped in gaining a healthier body. The main target audience of this diet is people who suffer from obesity. Make sure you consult your doctor on your health before you take on this diet. On to the benefits now:

• It helps you lose weight and perfect your figure.
• It prevents cardiovascular diseases by cutting down on your intake of fatty foods and excess calories.
• The diet also protects you from high blood pressure and cholesterol.
• Recipes are easy to understand.
• There are many programs online that make a customized diet according to your needs.
• You do not have to starve, but rather eat a meal rich in proteins.

The Biggest Loser diet stresses eating calories from vegetables and fruits, which will keep you healthy. It also mandates a food journal to keep count of your calorie intake and the various methods you follow to control yourself. It is a protein-rich diet, which makes you full and burns all your fat.

Important nutrients:

Some nutrients are essential in this weight loss program. They suck away the fat from the body and decrease the risk of cardiovascular disease. Here are some extremely important nutrients that are essential in this diet:

Proteins: Proteins are the building blocks of our cells, and they repair the tissues in our body. Proteins also help in reducing weight, which is why it made the list. Around 10-35% of our nutrients have to be proteins, which you can obtain by eating legumes, eggs, green vegetables, and so on.

Carbohydrates: They are the main source of energy for our body and especially beneficial to the brain. To maintain your intake of carbohydrates, you can eat grains like rice, fruits and vegetables, bread, and so on. These foods have a lot of fibers that decrease the risk of heart disease.

Calcium: It is a vital mineral that helps in strengthening the bones, muscle movement and maintaining blood flow. Yogurt and milk are rich sources of calcium.

Fat: Even though fat can be harmful to your health, you need certain types of fat that are important for our sustenance. It helps in absorbing essential vitamins like Vitamin A and D, among others. Around 20-35% of your food intake should have fats in it. Make sure you eat foods like fish and nuts to get omega-3 fats, which help in the development of your body. Do not consume fat-rich foods like meats.

It is important to get proper nutrient content to make sure your body functions properly. Make sure you choose your food carefully. Below is a chart on which foods are best for maintaining your health and how each helps.

Fruits:
Focus on fruits.
- Eat a variety of fruit.
- Chose fresh, frozen, canned or dried fruit.
- Go easy on fruit juices.

Vegetables:
Vary your veggies.
- Eat more green dark veggies.
- Eat more orange veggies.
- Eat more dry beans and peas.

Physical Activity
Find your balance between food & physical activity.
- Be physically active for 30 minutes most days of the week.
- Children and teenagers should be physically active for 60 minutes everyday or most days of the week.

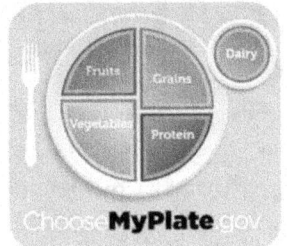

Oils:
Know your fats.
- Make most of your fat sources from fish, nuts and vegetable oils.
- Limit solid fats like butter, stick margarine, shortening, and lard.

Milk:
Get your calcium-rich foods.
- Go low-fat or fat-free
- If you don't or can't consume milk, chose lactose-free products or other calcium sources.

Grains:
Make at least half your grains whole.
- Eat at least 3 ounces of whole grain bread, cereal, rice, or pasta everyday.
- Look for the word "whole" before the grain name on the list of ingredients.

Meats & Beans
Go lean on protein.
- Choose low-fat or lean meats and poultry.
- Bake it, broil it or grill it.
- Vary your choices with more fish, beans, peas, nuts, and seeds.

Source: ChooseMyPlate.gov

14

Interesting facts:

Here are a few interesting facts about the Biggest Loser diet that might leave you shocked!

- It has the largest database of food, with up to 2,000,000 entries.
- You can eat until you are full; split your meals to 5-6 times a day!
- It was actually created by combining the principles of many other diets like Mediterranean, DASH, and TLC, among others.
- There are resorts that have programs based on this diet; they check your weight

and health and prepare a diet plan accordingly.

Tips to follow:
It is necessary to follow the diet you have chosen. Here are a few tips that can help you with your diet and exercise plan:

Nutrition is very, very important:
Make sure you consume a lot of nutrients. To do that, eat food like vegetables, fruits, and whole wheat grains that are rich in fibers and other nutrients. Make sure you have a journal to maintain records of your nutrition and calorie intake.

Reducing carbs will not help you:
Sometimes people think that just keeping away from carbs will help them lose weight. Giving up carbs is just one part of maintaining any diet. Exercising is also necessary if you want to maintain a healthy body.

Make sure you follow the diet: This diet requires a lot of sacrifices. This means you cannot indulge or eat whatever you want. You need to strictly follow the diet. It is not necessary to maintain the same diet plan; you can be creative with your recipes.

You can indulge once a week and eat junk food, but make sure you do not go overboard.

Do not starve yourself: Some people assume that starving and exercising will help them lose weight quickly. It is important you understand that starving does NOT help. It is important to have meals every 2-3 hours. Instead of starving yourself, you can skip dinner. This makes your body eat away the excess fat.

Talk to your trainer (if you plan on getting one): Make sure you inform your trainer if you feel you cannot handle the exercises. You cannot become slim in a day, and it takes time for you to learn these exercises and have the stamina to do them. Do not be afraid to look for a trainer who understands your condition. It is necessary for you to be comfortable with your trainer. It will only help you in your goal to lose weight.

RECIPES

Breakfast
Veggie Frittata with Turkey Bacon

Ingredients
- 1 packet low-fat turkey bacon
- 1 tablespoon of vegetable oil
- 1 cup green and red peppers, diced
- 1 cup mushrooms, chopped
- ½ cup asparagus, chopped
- 2 cups of eggs
- 1 cup milk
- 1/3 cup cheese
- 1 tablespoon of fresh parsley, diced
- 1/3 cup onions, chopped

Preparation
Pre-heat your oven at 350 degrees. Take a muffin tray and place the turkey bacon into the cups. Cook the turkey in the oven. While your turkey is cooking, heat oil over medium heat and add the peppers, asparagus and mushrooms.

Let cook for 5-6 minutes. Make sure your turkey is cooked and then cut them and place them on a plate.

Then, take a bowl and mix the eggs, parsley and milk. Put the bacon, cheese, onions and pepper mixture into a pan and stir. Put everything into the muffin cup and leave it in the oven for 20 minutes.

Lunch
Creamy Broccoli Pasta and Chicken

Ingredients
- 2 cups of broccoli, boiled
- 1 cup of basil leaves
- 4 garlic cloves, diced
- 2 tablespoons vegetable broth
- 2 teaspoons virgin olive oil
- 1-2 cups yogurt
- Seasoning (pepper, parmesan, salt)
- 4 pieces of chicken breast
- Olive oil
- Salt and pepper
- Pasta
- 18 cherry tomatoes, sliced

Preparation
Put the garlic, broccoli, parmesan and basil into a blender and whirl until roughly chopped. Pour oil and vegetable broth into the blender. Blend until the mixture is finely diced. Put the mixture in a bowl and stir with salt and yogurt.

Sprinkle in some pepper for added flavor. Prepare a grill, making sure you pre-heat it over high heat. Sprinkle a little olive oil on the chicken breasts and add salt and pepper. Place the breasts on the grill for 4-5 minutes on both sides.

Make sure your chicken is cooked properly and not pink on either side. Cook the pasta as instructed on the package.

Add the pasta to a large bowl, mix it with the broccoli mixture, and top it with cherry tomatoes. Place pasta and chicken on plate and serve.

Dinner
Waldorf Salad

Ingredients
- Cooked chicken breast
- 1 cup green and red apples, thinly sliced
- Celery
- Chopped walnuts
- Chopped onions
- 2 wedges of clementine
- 1 tablespoon fat-free Greek yogurt

Preparation

Dice the chicken breast. Add all your ingredients to a bowl and mix. Serve in lettuce cups or as is.

It is important for you to understand what the diet necessitates. You must be completely dedicated and strong willed to follow this diet. It is a long-term diet that requires you to give up fatty foods and follow a diet plan.
This is not for people who might have diseases that will aggravate if you vigorously exercise. Instead, you can make a plan suited to your health problems that might even help you rid yourself of them.

The workout has been proven to be very effective and healthy, but remember not to overdo it.

Chapter 7

Secrets about the Ornish Diet

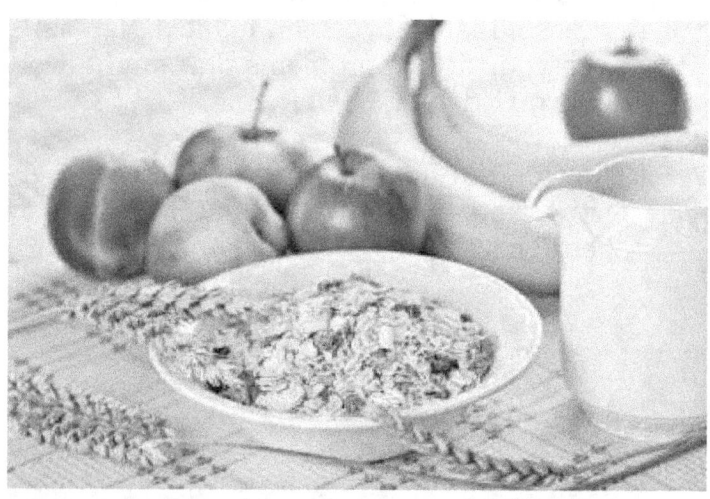

Diets usually give us a sinking feeling. After all, everyone wants to eat what they would like to. Fitness experts across the world claim that dieting can be fun. Before you reel back in shock, the status quo mandates that we transform our way of living.

We toast to a healthy life every year, right? Why don't we want to diet then? Maybe it's because diets are strict. They curb our sense of freedom.

Maybe that is not completely true.

In 2007, Dr. Dean Ornish released his book called "The Spectrum". This book covered all things diet-related: from exercise regimens to emotional sustenance options. In this book, he also wrote about fitness programs, the advantages of diets and the concept of healthy living. His book is considered to be a "book of diets", but what makes it so different from the rest?

It is simple: the fact that Dr. Ornish does not offer a severe routine to follow is what makes this diet appealing. He offers tips, solutions, and advice, and lists healthy foods and exercise patterns.

How you practice it is up to you.

#1. The Premise:

The US News and World Reports ranked the Ornish Diet as No.1 in 2012.

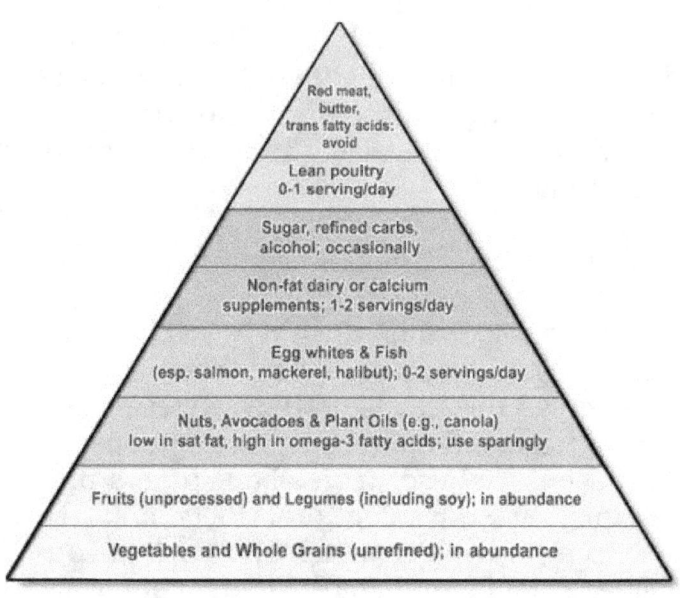

Red meat,
butter,
trans fatty acids:
avoid

Lean poultry
0-1 serving/day

Sugar, refined carbs,
alcohol; occasionally

Non-fat dairy or calcium
supplements; 1-2 servings/day

Egg whites & Fish
(esp. salmon, mackerel, halibut); 0-2 servings/day

Nuts, Avocadoes & Plant Oils (e.g., canola)
low in sat fat, high in omega-3 fatty acids; use sparingly

Fruits (unprocessed) and Legumes (including soy); in abundance

Vegetables and Whole Grains (unrefined); in abundance

In his book, Dr. Ornish classifies food into five categories based on how healthy they are. The list is arranged in descending order, from Most Healthy to Least Healthy. The first group consists of foods that are considered to be the healthiest of the categories, and this includes soy products, vegetables and fruits.

Needless to say, the food products listed in Group Five include extremely fatty food such as deep-fried food, egg yolks and red meat.

Starting off with this diet is quite simple.

Using Ornish's book, find out where you stand in the nutrition spectrum. This will be based on the foods you consume every day.

Then, decide on your objectives. This is most likely the toughest step, as you need to keep in mind your physical situation and motivation level.

The quantitative objectives are pretty simple to decide on; you will want to move to the top three food groups and start eating healthier foods.

If you have a health condition already and want to combat or treat it, then you will have to exert extra effort into your diet.

#2. How it works:

Dr. Ornish states that he released this book to help people combat diseases, while making sure that doing so doesn't make a dent in their wallet. Usually, doctor's check-ups and medical procedures leave us with a financial headache.

He emphasizes that your health is directly under your control. Therefore, you should be the one dictating what you should eat.

His book states the exact break-down of caloric intake, keeping different kinds of food in mind.

The diet breaks down the calories initially in this manner:

-       10% from fats
-       70% from carbohydrates
-       20% from proteins

What you do after that is decide how you want to stock your cupboards. The less healthy your supplies are, the more you need to compensate with exercise.

The Ornish diet has three parts to it, besides food items. Firstly, exercise. How much you exercise determines how fit you can be in the long run. Jogging, aerobics and resistance training are some activities it recommends.

Secondly, the diet insists on managing stress. Activities like meditation, yoga and deep breathing are recommended. Thirdly, Dr. Ornish emphasizes on spending time with your family, friends and relatives. This way, you have adequate emotional support, and this is said to reflect positively on your health in a lot of ways.

#3. How do I follow it?

Every diet calls for some mental preparation before starting off. The Ornish diet isn't bound by a book. Goals vary from person to person. If you are just looking to be fit, you have to follow a different regimen. If you already have a heart condition, then you need to buck up and take control of your lifestyle.

Here are some of the broad recommendations that can be followed:

-        Unless weight loss is at the top of your list, caloric intake is unrestricted. Now, this does not mean gorging on fries. The optimum daily caloric intake is 2,000 calories or less.

-        Trade in fatty red meat with heart-friendly food such as wild salmon. This helps in reducing your cholesterol.

-        Alcohol is generally discouraged, but one can have up to two ounces daily.

-        This diet suggests that you spread your meals in small portions every day. Recurrent, small-portioned meals can help you stay full. Moreover, they help maintain your energy levels.

-     Drop animal products, such as poultry and meat. They are high in cholesterol and saturated fats. Also, try to restrict your caffeine intake.

-     Make sure you limit your sugar intake to two servings a day. Salt intake should be less than 2,300 mg daily.
-     Consume ten percent or less of your calories from fat. Make sure that this fat is derived from unsaturated fats as much as possible.

-     It is found that whole grains, vegetables and fruits are all sources of fiber and "good" carbohydrates. Additionally, these help in keeping us full for longer periods of time.

#4. What the diet calls for:

This diet isn't one set in stone. It's highly individualistic, right from the objectives to the method of practice. It just prescribes certain guidelines, which are extremely flexible. The diet is meant to set meaningful standards for yourself so you can adopt them for life.

So, don't sweat if something goes wrong. We are human after all.

• Sometimes, we may just forget about our resolution and indulge, and that is okay. Make sure you compensate for it by eating healthier foods the next day.

• You may have overslept and missed your morning run. Make up for it the next day.

• Don't starve yourself just to lose some weight. This diet is not about straining yourself; instead, it is about choosing smaller portions of food initially. Practicing temperance in eating is important. Choose foods that are listed in the healthier end of the spectrum.

• As said before, the diet doesn't stop with just picking the right food. It is a synergy of exercise, healthy eating and mental stimulation. The diet was constructed to suit all individuals, so what you do to follow it is up to you.

• It is a "compassionate" diet. This is because the diet is one through which you can't fail. The diet doesn't prescribe any ultimatums. So, if you find yourself over-eating one day, make sure you eat healthy the next couple of days. It is as simple as that.

#5. What you see is what you get:

The Ornish diet embraces freedom, to say the least. You allow yourself to choose dieting plans and schedules. Still need more reasons to choose this diet?

Read on.
-        This diet is based on thirty-five years of research done by Dr. Dean Ornish. At the end of the research, it was found that following this diet helped reverse coronary heart disease. Medicare is even covering the dietary program due to its acclaimed success.

-        Dr. Ornish conducted an extensive study along with Nobel prize-winning Dr. Elizabeth Blackburn. This study proved that the Ornish diet helped improve telomerase levels by thirty percent.

Telomerase is a kind of enzyme that mends and elongates the ends of telomeres. These are a type of chromosomes and they determine how long we live.

-        The study conducted by Dr. Ornish involved 35 volunteers. Twenty of the thirty-five people had to follow a vegetarian diet, which was low-fat in nature. Egg whites were allowed once a day, as was one cup of non-fat milk. Cholesterol was curbed to just 5 mg daily. They had to practice stress managing techniques for an hour every day, exercise three hours a week, and attend group meetings twice a week.

-       It was seen that after a year, an average of twenty-four pounds of weight was lost. After five years, the participants maintained a twelve pound loss. Also, cardiac risks were reduced in some participants who had heart-related problems.

-       A result from the study showed that this diet helped in reducing the development of premature prostate cancer.

-       Many dietitians say that this diet is successful because it targets the right areas in our body. The Ornish diet helps in turning on genes that avert diseases, while turning off the genes that endorse colon, prostate and breast cancer. It was also noted that 500 genes were successfully benefited in just three months.

RECIPES

Breakfast
Spinach Egg-White Omelet

Ingredients
• 4-5 cherry tomatoes, halved or quartered
• 3 egg whites
• ½ cup onion, sliced or diced
• ½ cup spinach, roughly chopped
• Salt and Pepper, to taste

Preparation
• Sauté the onions for two to three minutes over medium heat.
• Add the spinach and cook for a few minutes.
• Once they are thoroughly cooked, crack three eggs and pour the whites over them.
• Add the seasoning and tomatoes. Cook the mixture by baking it at in the oven for 15-17 minutes at 350 Fahrenheit.
• Serve.

Lunch
Asian Noodle Salad with Peppers and Peanuts

Ingredients

For salad dressing:

Ingredients
- 3 garlic cloves, chopped
- 1 teaspoon sesame oil
- 2 teaspoon sugar
- ½ cup rice vinegar
- 2 tablespoon olive oil
- 2 teaspoon soy sauce

For salad:

Ingredients
- ½ packet spaghetti
- ½ cup peanuts
- ½ yellow bell pepper, finely sliced
- ½ red bell pepper, finely sliced
- ½ cup carrot, diced

Preparation
- Take all the dressing ingredients and mix them thoroughly.
- Let the mixture set for an hour, just to infuse the flavors together.
- Cook the vegetables and let sit for a while.

- Cook the noodles and let cool.
- Mix the noodles with the vegetables, once cooled.
- Mix the dressing once again. Add it to the noodle and vegetable mixture.
- Stir till they are combined, and serve.

Dinner

Bean & Spinach Whole-Wheat Pasta

Ingredients
- 450 grams whole-wheat pasta
- 500 grams white beans, rinsed
- ½ cup vegetable or chicken broth
- 2 garlic cloves, finely chopped
- 2 table spoon olive oil
- 300 grams spinach, roughly chopped
- ¼ cups bread crumbs, plain or seasoned

Preparation
- Cook the pasta in water for 10 minutes.
- While boiling, add a pinch of salt to the pasta.
- Toast breadcrumbs on a pan, after adding a tablespoon of olive oil. Toast for five minutes or so.

•   In another pan, add one tablespoon of oil and heat over medium heat. Sauté the garlic for half a minute.

•   Add the spinach and beans. Add the broth and cook for 3 minutes, or until the spinach is wilted.

•   Once the pasta is cooked, drain. However, keep some of the pasta water as reserve. Add the bean and spinach sauce to the pasta.

•   Simultaneously, stir in the reserve pasta water, tablespoon by tablespoon until the desired consistency is reached. Season with a pinch of salt.

•   Lightly sprinkle the pasta with breadcrumbs as garnish.

Chapter 8

Secrets about the Vegan Diet

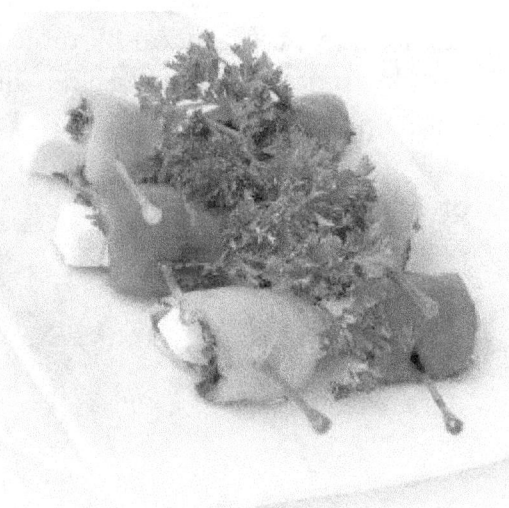

The vegan diet is one of the most popular diets these days. This diet helps in rapid weight loss as it focuses on consuming natural foods that are low in fat. It is a healthy choice, and this is why very few vegans are overweight. Unlike crash diets, this diet can be followed as a long-term practice.

You don't need to starve yourself; instead, you can have a high-fiber breakfast, a balanced meal for lunch and a light dinner. It is more popular among those who believe in animal rights and those who have dairy intolerance.

This diet came into limelight after former US president Bill Clinton revealed that he owed his weight loss to a plant-based diet.

Pop singer Beyonce lost around 65 pounds after coupling this diet with cardio workouts. She underwent a 22-day cleanse during which she had nothing but fruits, plants and snacks like cucumber.

Many elite athletes attribute their success to the vegan diet.

Claims and primary benefits

The vegan diet relies heavily on fruits and vegetables, which are low in calories and make you feel full quickly, though the calorie intake is small. This diet is high in fiber, cancer-fighting antioxidants and complex carbohydrates. The amount of saturated fat consumed on this diet is small. Hence, it leads to rapid weight loss without having to starve the body. This diet will also make sure that the cholesterol and blood pressure levels are maintained. It also prevents heart problems, cancer and other chronic diseases.

What to include in the diet?

The vegan diet is purely a plant-based diet that consists of fruits, vegetables, seeds, nuts, whole grains, legumes and leafy greens. Eat a variety of fruits and vegetables to maintain a balanced diet, but no poultry, meat or fish is allowed.

It is quite like the vegetarian diet, except for the fact that this diet does not allow animal products like eggs, dairy or honey either! Refined carbs are off limits, and vegans also do not consume foods that are refined using animal products, such as wine and refined sugar. Caffeine and alcohol are strictly prohibited on this diet. Sodas or even diet sodas are also not allowed.

Additional Benefits

This diet is great for your skin, as avoiding dairy products is believed to be beneficial to your skin. It can change your acne-prone skin into shiny, clear skin overnight. Those who switch to a vegan diet also report to have better quality of sleep.

It also reduces aging effects. Additionally, the cost incurred while following this diet is less compared to many other diets, since costly food like red meat is cut down.

Facts

But you have to be careful while following this diet. Nutrients like protein, iron, calcium, vitamin B12, vitamin D and omega-3 are not provided in this diet. It is better to consult a physician first. Utmost care has to be taken to see that all the nutrients are provided for pregnant women and children following this diet.

But on the other hand, the amount of saturated fat consumed on this diet is very small, so it is easy to keep cholesterol and blood pressure under check. It prevents heart disease, cancer and other chronic diseases. It is not the amount of calories that matter for weight loss. What matters is the sources from which those calories are obtained. Since the calories in this diet come from natural sources, it is easier to burn them away.

Proteins- Plants do not provide adequate amount of protein required by the body, so it is better to include cereals and pulses.

Iron- The iron obtained from cereals, pulses and tofu is less absorbed by the body than iron obtained from animal products. For better absorption of iron, Vitamin C is required. Also, the intake of tea should be reduced as it slows down the absorption process.

Iodine- It is a special component of the thyroid hormones and plays a vital role in growth, metabolism and the functioning of the key organs. This diet may not offer enough iodine, and hence, vegans are under the risk of suffering from deficiency or even goitre.

Calcium- Calcium is vital for bone growth and for the teeth. Lack of calcium will lead to osteoporosis and weakening of bones. Since the vegan diet prohibits dairy products, those following the diet should consume almond milk or soy milk. Citrus fruits and vegetables like cabbage and broccoli are also good sources of calcium.

Vitamin D- It is necessary for vegans to get plenty of this essential nutrient. Vitamin

D is found in cereals, yogurts and mush-rooms. Supplements are also available.

Vitamin B12- This is required for the vital functioning of the red blood cells. Vitamin B12 is not found in plants. To meet this requirement, yeast, soya or vitamin supplements can be taken.

Omega-3- Plant oils, almonds, walnuts and hazelnuts will compensate for the absence of fish in the diet. They have to be taken regularly.

Zinc- Zinc is an important component of the enzymes. As in the case of iron, zinc is easily absorbed from animal sources rather than plant sources. Sources of zinc include whole grains, nuts, legumes and soy products.

Additional tips

It is difficult to switch to veganism all of a sudden. The transition should take place gradually. Try cutting down meat from your meals one by one, replacing it with a vegan substitute.

For example, you could replace chicken with tofu. You might be tempted to go back to eating red meat if you see someone having it around you. So have a good group of friends who support you. Motivate each

other, and try different vegan dishes together. Check out if there are any interesting
vegan restaurants in your neighborhood.

RECIPES

Breakfast
Cabbage-O-Mania

Ingredients
- 1 cabbage, chopped
- 1 onion, sliced
- Olive oil
- Garlic powder
- Salt
- Pepper

Preparation
Chop the cabbage into large chunks. Steam the cabbage until the white parts of the cabbage become clear. Heat the olive oil in a separate pan. Sauté the onions until they become soft and golden brown. Add garlic powder, pepper and salt to the onions. Stir the mixture thoroughly, then stir in the cabbage. Enjoy!

Lunch
Moroccan Stew

Ingredients
- Chickpeas
- 2 tomatoes, chopped
- 2 carrots, chopped

- 1 onion, diced
- 1 parsnip, chopped
- 1 teaspoon cumin
- 1 teaspoon mild chili powder
- Coriander
- 1 sachet of lemon & coriander couscous
- 2 tablespoons tomato purée
- Olive oil

Preparation

Chop the tomatoes, onion and carrots. Sauté the chopped carrots, chopped onion and the chopped parsnips for ten minutes in olive oil. Sprinkle the cumin and chili powder over the vegetables. Then, add the chopped tomatoes, the chickpeas and the purée. Pour some boiling water in the empty tomato can until half full, then swirl it and pour it into the stew. Season with salt and pepper. Then allow it to simmer for 20 minutes or until the vegetables are soft and cooked thoroughly. Make the couscous by following the instructions on the packet, and serve it with the stew once it is cooked. Serve with yogurt.

Snack
Potato wedges

Ingredients
- 2 potatoes
- Olive oil

- Salt to taste

Preparation

Heat the oven at 392 Fahrenheit. Wash the potatoes. Do not remove the peel off the potatoes. Wipe them dry with kitchen paper, then chop into large wedges to get 4 to 6 pieces per potato. Dry the pieces again with kitchen paper. Mix some oil and salt and put them in a large freezer bag. Add the wedges inside the freezer bag and shake to coat. Now place the wedges in a shallow braking tray. Bake for 30-40 minutes until they turn golden brown and look crispy. Your yummy potato wedges are ready to be served. Serve with mayonnaise or tomato ketchup.

Dinner
Sautéed Kale

Ingredients
- 1 teaspoon olive oil
- 1 onion, sliced
- 1 garlic clove, crushed
- 1/4 cup of water
- 1 bunch of kale, chopped
- 1 tomato, diced

Preparation

In an iron skillet mix oil, onion and garlic. Add water. Cook the mixture over medium heat until the onions become transparent, then add kale. Saute for 5 minutes or until the kale wilts. Add tomato to the mixture. Cook until the tomato releases its juice. Your sautéed kale is ready. Serve it hot.

The Vegan diet is one of the diets you can choose for weight loss. It can be integrated into your lifestyle to make it a healthy one. By following this diet, you can expect rapid weight loss. This diet also requires physical exercise for a minimum of 30 minutes per day. Now you can realize your dream of having that beach body with this low-fat diet. The Vegan diet also keeps your skin glowing. Plus, it keeps the cholesterol and blood pressure levels under check. It also prevents heart problems and other chronic diseases.

Chapter 9

Secrets about the DASH Diet

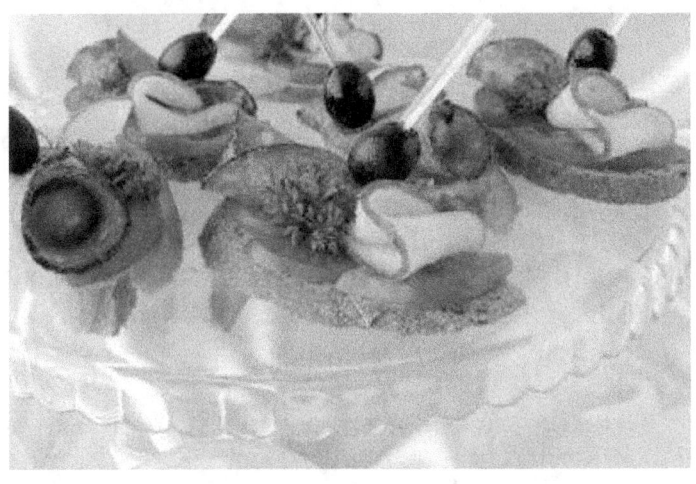

Physical well-being is vital for mental well-being. The DASH diet was incepted by the US National Institutes of Health, and the primal focus was to help reduce the risk of hypertension.

Soon enough, this diet proved to be an all-star. An acronym for Dietary Approaches to Stop Hypertension, the DASH diet has been ranked #1 for the past four years by various wellness institutes and websites.

This being said, the diet focuses on the blanket concept of healthy eating. It emphasizes on consuming the right kind of food so high blood pressure can be avoided.

This acclaimed diet has thousands of followers who indisputably testify its success.

Claims of the diet:

Primarily, this diet focuses on reducing the danger of hypertension. High blood pressure and high cholesterol cause many health complications. Potassium, calcium, and magnesium are the core nutrients that help lower blood pressure.

The diet isn't bound by time. It mandates a lifestyle change, coupled with careful moderation of what you eat. The diet focuses on reducing sodium intake and helps one substitute it with less harmful nutrients.

The daily regimen requires you to carefully track what you eat. A proper diet can help in curbing the risk of various other diseases such as osteoporosis, stroke and diabetes etc.

Although the diet doesn't list weight loss as its priority, following the diet ensures that you shed off excess pounds.

This diet emphasizes on eating fruits, vegetables and low-fat dairy. This can be coupled with adequate amounts of lentils, nuts, poultry, fish and whole grains.

<u>There are three variations of the diet itself:</u>

Standard diet:

While following this diet, you are allowed to consume a maximum of 2,300 mg of sodium daily.

Lower Sodium DASH diet:

This diet is followed by those who already suffer from conditions such as high blood pressure and diabetes. If you are over 51 years of age, then it's time for you to be extra careful about your sodium intake.

Weight-loss DASH diet:

As stated before, weight loss is not the primary aim of this diet. If indeed weight loss is your aim, you can also set a daily caloric goal of 1,600. Usually, the DASH diet works on a daily caloric count of 2,000.

This is one of the major benefits of the DASH diet; you can tailor it according to individual circumstances, without many serious repercussions.

The Dietary Guidelines for Americans says that the average amount of sodium intake is 3,500 mg per day. So, following this diet helps keep your sodium levels under check.

What to eat?

The DASH diet consists of vegetables, whole grains, and a variety of legumes, fruits, poultry and fish. This diet is fool-proof, as it recommends items that have low saturated fat and little cholesterol.

A day on this diet would typically consist of the following:
Vegetables:

Servings: 4-5 daily

Pick vegetables such as carrots, sweet potatoes and other green, leafy vegetables. These vegetables are rich in magnesium, fiber and vitamins.

One serving would include 1 cup of raw vegetables, in the case of leafy vegetables. You can have half a cup of chopped raw or steamed vegetables.

Fruits:

Servings: 4- 5daily

Fruits are as essential to this diet as vegetables are. Pick fruits with low sugar content. A single serving can be: a medium-sized fruit, 120 ml of fresh fruit juice or ½ cup of canned fruit. In the case of canned fruit, make sure no sugar is added.

Dairy products:

Servings: 2-3 daily

Saturated fat is the main reason for having high cholesterol, which makes you more susceptible to heart disease. Most dairy products have large amounts of saturated fat. Yet, they are rich in calcium and protein.

While following this diet, ensure that you pick non-fat or low-fat dairy products. Cheese should be avoided as much as possible. Even fat-free cheeses have high sodium content.

Daily Nutritional Goals in the DASH diet (for a 2,000-C

Total fat	27% of calories
Saturated fat	6% of calories
Protein	18% of calories
Carbohydrate	55% of calories
Cholesterol	150 mg
Sodium	2,300 mg*
Potassium	4,700 mg
Calcium	1,250 mg
Magnesium	500 mg
Fiber	30 g

http://www.medi
calnew-

Poultry, fish and meat:

Servings: 6 or less daily

Fish is a safer option for your heart than poultry. Likewise, opt to eat turkey rather than duck or goose. Lean meat also has high cholesterol content. What this diet emphasizes is healthy food choices. So, cut back on your meat portions and add vegetables instead. When you choose to eat meat, make sure that you boil or grill it, rather than frying. A serving would include around 31 grams of meat or seafood, or a single egg.

#3. The results say:

A panel of over 39 fitness experts and dietitians chose 48 subjects to test the efficiency of this diet. A 28-day diet plan was formulated for the participants to follow.

After this, it was seen that:
1) Patients with pre-hypertension had an average drop of 6 mm Hg and 3 mm Hg in systolic and diastolic pressure.

2) Subjects who had hypertension experienced a fall in systolic pressure by 11 mm Hg and diastolic pressure by 6 mm Hg.

3) These significant changes were seen without any weight reduction.

4) Cholesterol levels were ideal, as the individuals were subjected to a balanced diet.

A major revelation in 2013 showed that following this diet also helps in curbing many complications that lead to kidney stone formation. Therefore, this diet keeps obesity, blood pressure and kidney stones in check.

#4. How does it work?

Four medical centers, aided by the NHLBI, conducted two DASH studies. In the first one, 459 adults were engaged. In this pool, it was seen that 27% had high blood pressure. Half the participants were female and 60% of the participants were African-American. Three diet plans were compared. The first one was that followed by average Americans. The second plan was like the first, except it had more fruits and vegetables. The third one was the DASH menu.

All these plans had an average sodium content of 3,000 mg each day. By the end of two weeks, it was seen that the blood pressure of participants following the DASH menu had fallen. Also, these participants were more fit and active.

The second study concentrated more on sodium intake and its correlation with blood pressure.

A total of 412 participants were randomly assigned one of two menus, with three different sodium levels. These levels were monitored for a month. The highest intake was 3,300 mg per day, followed by 2,300 mg per day and the lowest intake of 1,500 mg per day. With the fall in sodium intake, there was a corresponding fall in blood pressure. The greatest fall was seen in the last menu.

The working of the DASH diet is ingenious and specific. By reducing sodium intake, the chances of high blood pressure are prevented. The diet is also precautionary in nature. The diet calls for the intake of magnesium; potassium and calcium to help regulate blood pressure.

By reducing the intake of saturated fat, one is no longer susceptible to high cholesterol. This also helps prevent heart disease. Although losing weight isn't the goal, the diet is tailored to help reduce excess fat and maintain a healthy level of blood pressure.

#5. How do I cope with the diet?

Settling into a new pattern can be tough. The DASH diet plan comes with dozens of e-books, pamphlets and recipe ideas.

Here are a few tips you can turn to, when in need:

• Fat-free milk has just 80 calories. Plus, it has no fat. Fat-free milk is especially used to help lower blood pressure.

• Experiment with salads. Use quinoa, chickpeas and other beans to lighten up your salad. Use an array of vegetables. You can season them, but go easy on the packaged spices.

• Next time you're craving for a creamy dip, go for a low-fat dip such as hummus. Also, you can stir-fry the vegetables. This way, you won't get bored!

• Think minimal meat. Pick heart-friendly fish like salmon over poultry and meat. More so, try to cut down the servings of meat after each day. Replace meat with different kinds of vegetables and tofu.

• This diet has no restriction on canned vegetables or fruits. Make sure that the label says "No added salt" and "No added preservatives".

• A good way to integrate weight-loss and DASH is to replace usual sources of carbohydrates with substitutes. For example, eat whole-wheat noodles and brown rice now and then.

RECIPES

Breakfast
Quinoa Breakfast Bowl

Ingredients
- 2 cups of cooked quinoa
- 340 grams of boiled and cut broccoli
- 285 grams of thawed spinach
- A small bowl of cheddar cheese
- Onion powder
- Garlic powder
- Black pepper
- Low salt seasoning
- Dozen eggs
- Low salt, organic salsa
- Nutmeg

Preparation
1. Put the eggs in a bowl with cold water and add salt to them.
2. Boil them on a medium flame.
3. Let them boil for 5-6 minutes if you prefer soft boiled eggs or 10 minutes for hard boiled eggs.
4. Put some ice or cold water into the bowl and pour out the hot water.

5. Let them sit till they have cooled.
6. Peel the eggs, a small tip would be to wet your fingers before to peel them easily.
7. Then, take a large mixing bowl and add your quinoa, broccoli, spinach, spices, a dash of nutmeg and finally the cheese.
8. Mix the ingredients till it is uniformly spread.
9. Taste and check your seasoning.
10. Add more if you need to.

Lunch
Honey Citrus Chicken and Spinach

Ingredients
1. **Chicken**
- Deboned chicken breast
- ¼ teaspoon of salt
- ½ teaspoon of black pepper
- Vinegar
- 2 tablespoons of whole wheat flour
- Olive oil
- Orange
- 1 cup white wine
- 2 tablespoons of diet honey
2. **Spinach**

- One packet of spinach
- Cut onions
- 3 cloves of finely chopped garlic
- 1 ½ teaspoon of balsamic vinegar

Preparation
Chicken
- Place a pan with a bit of olive oil at medium flame.
- As your pan heats, wash your chicken breasts with a bit of vinegar and salt.
- Take a bowl and pour 2 tablespoons of whole wheat flour, ¼ tablespoon of salt and ½ teaspoon of black pepper and mix.
- Coat your chicken with this mixture and place it in the heated pan.
- Leave the chicken for three minutes on both sides.
- Take a bowl and add low sodium chicken broth and flour. Mix well.
- Pour it into a pan and add 1 cup white wine and 2 tablespoons of diet honey.
- Continue mixing; add orange zest and juice from an orange.
- Let it come to a boil and then add cinnamon sticks for flavor.

- Leave it for 3 minutes and place the chicken breast into the sauce.
- Leave it for three more minutes and your chicken is ready!

Spinach
- Put 1 tablespoon of olive oil into a saucepan.
- Heat it at medium flame.
- Add chopped onions and stir it until there is some color on the onions.
- Add 3 chopped cloves of garlic and finally add the spinach.
- The last ingredient to put in is 1 1/2 teaspoon of balsamic vinegar to give it a salty taste.
- You can add herbs to give an added flavor.

Dinner
Pappardelle with Lemon Gremolata and Asparagus

Ingredients
- 2 tablespoons of freshly sliced parsley
- 1 teaspoon of lemon zest
- 1 finely chopped clove of garlic
- 226 grams of pappardelle
- 226 grams of thinly cut asparagus

- 1/3 cup of cream (heavy)
- 1/2 teaspoon of salt
- 1/8 teaspoon of pepper

Preparation
- First, we need to make gremolata.
- Take a small bowl and add the diced parsley, garlic and lemon zest.
- Leave it aside and take a large saucepan.
- Add the pasta and cook. You can make your own pasta too.
- When the pasta is half cooked, add the asparagus.
- Drain it and wash with cold water. Keep it aside.
- Heat the saucepan; add cream, salt and pepper.
- Add the pasta to the pan and mix thoroughly.
- Cook cream until it thickens and stir continuously.
- Cook for about 3 minutes and add ¾ of the gremolata to the mixture.
- Cook for a minute and then top with remaining gremolata.

Chapter 10

Secrets about the Traditional Asian Diet

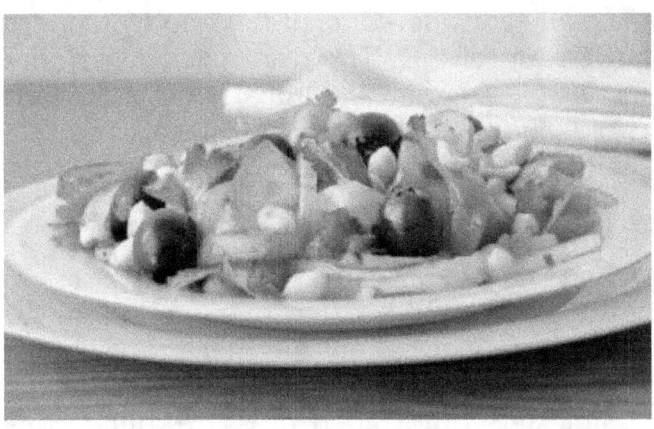

There are various diets that help in weight loss, and each diet has its own advantages and limitations. One of the best diets is the simple traditional Asian diet, which emphasizes low-fat food and is therefore very healthy. It has various options in the menu to suit one's liking.

The traditional Asian diet has rice, noodles, bread, whole grains, fruits, legumes, vegetables and nuts. It is a balanced diet that provides all the required nutrients to the body, unlike other diets.

Claims and primary benefits

It prevents a lot of diseases. Asians have lower rates of diseases like cancer, obesity and heart disease. That is why Asians are usually considered healthier and live longer than Americans. The traditional Asian diet is a low-fat diet and thus helps in weight loss. Another plus is that it makes you feel fuller and keeps hunger at bay.

Additional benefits

The foods in the Asian diet are low in fat and high in fiber, as the diet primarily focuses on fruits and vegetables. It keeps cholesterol and blood pressure under control and prevents heart disease, while also helping in the prevention and control of diabetes. To top it all off, this diet is said to have no side effects.

How does the diet work?

Asians consume rice, noodles, bread, whole grains, millets, fruits, vegetables, legumes, nuts and seeds. Fish and dairy are optional. Red meat can be consumed once a month. Eggs and poultry can be eaten once a week. A person on this diet must drink 6 glasses of water a day. Wine and beer can be consumed in moderation. It is okay to have something sweet once a week.

The Asian diet pyramid consists of daily physical activity at the bottom, and foods such as fruits, vegetables and legumes that are to be consumed daily are at the top. Since fish, shellfish and dairy are optional, they are second to bottom. Above them are eggs, poultry and sweets that are to be consumed on a weekly basis. And on the top of the pyramid is the red meat that can be consumed on a monthly basis. Indulge yourself in physical exercise for a minimum of 30 minutes a day.

The Asian diet is balanced because foods with various nutrients are consumed. Eating foods with specific nutrients might lead a person to the consequences of having too much of that nutrient. At the same time, he faces the risk of missing out on the other nutrients.

So this diet is flexible and not structured. You can plan what you eat and plan your exercise routine accordingly. Cost incurred on this diet is moderate, though preparing these dishes may take some effort.

Facts and figures

Calories alone don't matter. It is important to focus on where those calories come from. Asians consume around 25-40% more calories than Americans, and they still tend to be less obese. This is because they get more calories from natural sources that are easy to burn, and fewer calories from fat. They tend to release energy at a steady rate. But foods like artificial sweeteners, sodas, cookies and snacks spike the blood sugar level. Thus, they make you hungrier.

The Asian diet helps you to stick to the government's recommendation of 20-35% of daily calories from fat.

It provides around 16% of protein, which is well within the 10-35% range suggested by the government.

Anywhere between 45-65% of your daily calorie intake should be from carbohydrates. This diet provides 50%.

The recommended salt intake is 2,300 milligrams. If you are 50 years or older, or if you have diabetes or hypertension, the recommended intake is 1,500 milligrams or less.

Fiber is said to help digestion and make you think you are full. Recommended consumption of fiber is 22 to 34 grams. Since vegetables, fruits and whole grains are a major part of the diet, it can meet this recommendation easily.

What to eat on the diet?

The key food in the Asian diet is rice. It is better to have brown rice while following this diet than white rice. Brown rice is nothing but white rice with the surrounding husk. It is not refined, so the body makes a lot of effort to break down the outer shell, using up a lot of energy.

Another important part of this diet is the vegetables. It is better to have cooked vegetables than raw ones. Cooking the vegetables will destroy a small part of their nutrients, which reduces the load on the stomach during the digestion process. This makes it easier to send the good nutrients to the tissues and to send the wastes for excretion.

While following this diet, red meat should be consumed in reasonable amounts. Too much of it can lead to health problems, and at the same time, consuming very little red meat will cause long-term protein deficiency.

The traditional Asian diet suggests that it is best to stay away from dairy products. Dairy products do have calcium, but they also have a protein called Casein, which robs the bones of calcium. Green leafy vegetables, soy products and nuts are better sources of calcium, with fewer ill effects. Dairy also turns into phlegm, which can be present in the body as mucus, sinus infection, fat, skin conditions, fibroids and tumors. If necessary, low-fat dairy products can be consumed in moderate amounts.

It's suggested that you reduce coffee consumption as well while following the Asian diet. Instead, drink large quantities of water. Another good alternative is green tea, which is good for health, as it is said to prevent chronic diseases such as throat, lung, stomach and breast cancer.

For cooking, the Asian diet uses vegetable oils, which have unsaturated fats, whereas Western diets use butter and saturated fats. Saturated fat can lead to chronic diseases, so replacing saturated fats with unsaturated fats by using canola oil and olive oil can prevent heart disease.

Additional tips

When you follow the Asian diet, it is not necessary to take supplements since it is a balanced diet. Do not take sugar substitutes. The Asian diet suggests it is better to consume less processed foods.It is necessary to stay physically active while on this diet. Exercise for a minimum of 30 minutes per day. The diet suggests that you sleep for 7 hours a day. Take some time off work to re-energize yourself. After all, you have to be happy to be healthy. Home-made Asian foods are the best. Asian restaurants tend to deep fry and add sugary and starchy sauces to their dishes.

RECIPES

Breakfast
Mixed Vegetable Salad

Ingredients
- 1 tablespoon tomatoes, chopped
- 1 tablespoon celery
- 2-3Lettuce
- 1 tablespoon radishes, chopped
- 1 tablespoon carrots
- Pepper (as required)
- Pea shoots (as required)
- Cucumber, sliced (as required)
- Spring onion, sliced (as required)

Preparation
Wash the radishes, carrots, spring onion, celery and let
tuce until they are clean. Chop the tomatoes, radishes and cucumbers into small pieces. Peel the skin from the spring onion and chop it into pieces. Next, chop the celery. Put all of these ingredients together and mix them in a bowl. Your salad is now ready to be munched on!

Lunch
Tomato Sardine Risotto

Ingredients

- 140 grams risotto rice
- 500-600 grams vegetable stock (boiling hot)
- 1 can chopped tomatoes
- 1 red onion, chopped
- 2 garlic cloves, chopped
- 1 can of sardines (in tomato sauce)
- 1 red pepper, chopped
- Handful of peas
- Drops of lemon juice
- 1 teaspoon of paprika
- Grated cheese

Preparation

Fry the chopped red onion, chopped red pepper and garlic together for 5 minutes. Then add the risotto rice and paprika and fry mixture again for another 5 minutes. After that, add the chopped tomatoes and a splash of stock and allow the mixture to simmer on medium heat. Keep stirring the mixture until the rice absorbs all the liquid. Add more stock before repeating this again. When half the stock is gone, add the peas, sardines and drops of lemon juice. Continue to add the stock and wait for it to be absorbed until all the stock has gone. The rice should be well cooked. Serve with grated cheese and lots of pepper.

Snack

Rice Tikkis

Ingredients
- Rice
- 1 onion, finely chopped
- 1 ginger, finely chopped
- 1 garlic, finely chopped
- Green chillies, finely chopped
- Coriander
- Salt, to taste
- Chickpea flour
- Olive oil

Preparation
Mix the rice, chopped onion, chopped ginger, chopped garlic, chillies and coriander leaves in a bowl. Make small patties from the mixture. Add some olive oil in a pan and shallow fry the patties. Your rice tikka is ready to be served. Serve with some green chutney.

Dinner
Cheesy Chicken Pasta

Ingredients
- Pasta (any type)
- Pasta sauce
- 1 garlic, finely chopped
- 1 large onion, thinly sliced
- Sausages (if preferred)

- Mashed chicken
- 1 capsicum, finely chopped
- Grated cheese

Preparation
Cook the pasta in boiling water. Add salt to it. Fry the sausages and the mashed chicken separately in a different pan. Then, fry the finely chopped garlic, thinly sliced onion and finely chopped capsicum separately. While frying this mixture, reduce the heat and add the pasta, sausages and mashed chicken. Add sauce to it until it appears to have a soft red color. Sprinkle some grated cheese on it and the pasta is ready to be served hot!

Since the Asian diet takes more calories from natural sources, it does not store fat, making it easier to burn. This diet coupled with the right amount of exercise can help in weight loss while preventing a lot of chronic diseases.

Chapter 11

Secrets about the Jenny Craig Diet

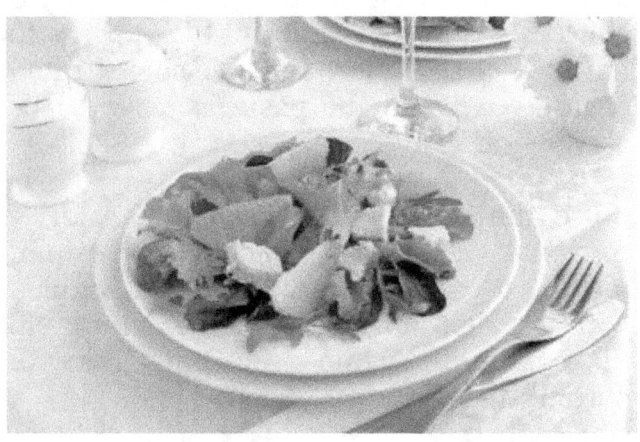

Jenny Craig Co. is a weight loss and well-ness firm established in 1983. The reason for its ever increasing popularity is its fa-mous diet plan. This plan is specially designed for each person who signs up.

Calorie intake is monitored by prescription of an appropriate amount of pre-packaged food by the company. This is a unique concept, as the chances of succumbing to tempting, calorie loaded food are slim.

You work with a personal consultant who not only decides your meals, but also plans your activity schedule. It is usually for half an hour for five days a week.

But is it the right diet plan for you? Read on to know some of the lesser known facts about the Jenny Craig diet.

The way it works

This a program meant for those who are aiming for a significant amount of weight loss in a stipulated time period. Your consultant will work with you to achieve your goal. The program is divided into two levels. The first level lasts until you are halfway to your target weight. While on this level, you eat pre-packaged meals prepared by Jenny Craig Co. according to your height, weight and target weight loss. You also have to follow a regular physical activity plan. After the first level is over, you have more or less acquainted yourself with the kind of food you need to eat and the size of the portions. So, in the second level, you are advised on how to prepare Jenny Craig meals at home.

This diet works on the principle of satiety. The Jenny Craig meals are balanced and don't completely cut off particular nutrients like fats or carbohydrates; they are just taken in limited amounts. In fact, the calories are derived from different nutrients of the meal in the proportion prescribed by American standards. Also, no foods are out of bounds. Alcohol and desserts are allowed, but in moderation. You usually have three meals and two or three snacks per day. Apart from that, you can eat unlimited fruits and non-starchy vegetables.

Convenient

In fact, convenient would be an understatement. This program is designed such that you can integrate this new meal plan smoothly into your busy life. In the first level, there is no need to prepare any food. Imagine how much time and effort it will save! In fact, you can get your food delivered to your doorstep. What's better than yummy food arriving home every time you feel hungry? Apart from this, your personal consultant will work with you to schedule your exercise plan. You can even change it every week according to your convenience. You also have online and telephone support 24/7. You have optional weekly sessions with your consultant as well to check your progress.

Not accommodative

Though it is a customized plan, this diet works usually the same way for everyone. It seems the only things taken into account are the height and weight of a person. For example, if you are a vegan or lactose intolerant, you won't find much variety in the Jenny Craig menu. Most of the packaged foods are meat-based. Even the vegetarian dishes are supplemented with milk and dairy products to ensure consumption of an apt amount of proteins. Also, if you want to go nutrient specific like gluten-free or low-sodium, there aren't much options. You might end up designing a plan for your preference, but it is quite tricky. This is a major setback, as they don't have these alternative meals in place.

Not in everyone's budget

The awesomeness, convenience and customization of this plan come at a huge price. Though the exact costs incurred vary from country to country and also within the US, it is safe to say that following this plan will create a big hole in your wallet. The initial registration fee is about $400, and the monthly registration fee is anything from $20 to $50, but they don't usually allow registration for less than 6 months. Apart from this, the pre-packaged Jenny Craig food costs about $15 to $20 per day. The high cost of this diet has so far kept most people from trying it.

Additional benefits

There are bound to be some brownie points when you are eating right and exercising too. Apart from losing that extra chunk of weight, you can benefit by getting expert advice from qualified nutritionists on your personal health issues. The diet plan is known to have great impact on the improvement of the cardiovascular system. It also helps prevent and control diabetes. In fact, they have a special plan for people with Type 2 diabetes. All of these facts are backed by studies conducted from time to time by the company as well as independently.

With all this information at hand, you can review and decide whether this diet plan is meant for you or not. Keep in mind your specific requirements and timeline before deciding. You can even drop by one of the company's centers for a consultation. If you do plan on following this diet, let us have a look at the kind of food you will be eating while on it. Though you don't need to cook much while on the first level, let us give you a head start with a peek at these absolutely delightful second level recipes from the Jenny Craig menu.

RECIPES

Breakfast
One of the classics for the first meal of the day - Mediterranean scrambled eggs

Ingredients
- 1 red onion, finely chopped
- ½ cup each of chopped zucchini, baby spinach and red capsicum
- 2 teaspoons of olive oil
- 4 eggs
- Chopped parsley (and some for garnishing)
- Worcestershire sauce
- Cracked black pepper

Preparation

Heat the oil in a pan. Add onion and capsicum and sauté them for some time. Now add zucchini and baby spinach and stir thoroughly. Beat the eggs and mix them with parsley, sauce and pepper. Make sure the sautéed vegetables are not too moist. Pour the mixture over the vegetables and mix thoroughly. Stir until the eggs are cooked. Garnish with parsley and your yummy eggs are ready.

Lunch
Something light, yet filling for lunch - Vegetable stir-fry with prawns and cashew

Ingredients
- 6 cups of assorted veggies, chopped
- 3 spring onions, sliced length-wise
- 1 fresh chili and 1 garlic clove, finely chopped
- 1 teaspoon ginger, grated
- Some coriander, chopped
- 1 spoonful low-sodium oyster sauce
- 2 spoonfuls low-sodium soy sauce
- 3 spoonfuls low-sodium vegetable stock
- 1 spoonful olive oil
- ¼ cup cashew nuts
- ½ kilograms raw prawns, peeled and with the tail intact

Preparation

Put the assorted veggies, spring onion and coriander in a mixing bowl. Add garlic, ginger and chilli and toss to combine. Heat a wok on the stove. Add olive oil and half the vegetable stock to it. Add the prawns when the wok is steaming and cook them for a few minutes. Add the veggies and stir-fry until the prawns turn pink, or until they reach your preferred doneness. You can add more stock now if needed. Top with cashew nuts and you are good to go.

Dinner

Try this exotic and spicy, yet healthy dish for dinner - Moroccan lemon chicken with green olives.

Ingredients

- 1 onion, finely diced
- ½ cup green olives
- 1 spoonful lemon skin
- 2 baby fennel, finely sliced
- ¼ liter low-sodium chicken broth
- 1 spoonful each of ground coriander and cinnamon
- 1 cinnamon stick
- 2 spoonfuls ground cumin
- ½ spoonful each of paprika and turmeric
- 2 spoonfuls olive oil
- ¾ kilograms chicken thighs (fat removed)

Preparation

Preheat your oven to 180C. Mix the fennel,

cinnamon stick, onion, lemon and olives. Spread the mixture in a big baking dish and put the chicken stock in it. Meanwhile, mix the oil and spices and marinate the chicken with this mixture. Add the chicken on top of the stock and roast for about 30 minutes. Now change the oven temperature to 200C and cook until the chicken is golden (about 20 minutes). Spicy chicken is ready to be savored!

Does it really look like dieting? Who wouldn't fall for these oh-so-delicious dishes on the Jenny Craig menu? And there's so much more! You will end up becoming a great cook after finishing the second level.

Overall, Jenny Craig is a great program to harness your weight and keep it under control, provided you keep yourself motivated and have the bucks. And while on the journey, you educate yourself about health and the right foods to eat, and start living a healthier lifestyle as a result. Hope you enjoy your experience with the Jenny Craig program.

Chapter 12

Secrets about the Mayo Clinic Diet

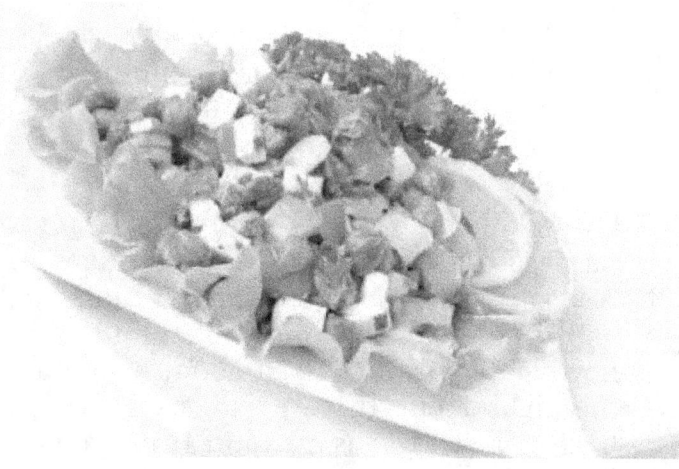

"Mayo Clinic Diet" - this phrase has been in vogue for quite a time. Many diets ranging from a grapefruit diet to a cabbage diet have been called the "Mayo Clinic Diet". They have been passed around by word of mouth and on the internet for decades. But the real version was announced and popularized by Mayo Clinic only recently. They also published a book about the diet - The Mayo Clinic Diet.

Let's us look at some of the little known facts about this amazing diet plan.

The way it works

According to Mayo Clinic, this diet is not a diet per se, but a way of life. It is primarily aimed at losing weight through adoption of healthy life habits. It is actually divided into two phases - 'Lose it' for the first two weeks and 'Live it' for the rest of your life. This diet works on the principle that you don't have to give up food, just modify your eating habits to include healthy and low-calorie options. Satiety of hunger is the main stay of this diet, and this is why it is much more doable than the other diets.

In the 'Lose it' phase, it concentrates on adopting 5 healthy habits and breaking 5 unhealthy habits. The healthy habits are eating a healthy breakfast, eating at least seven servings of vegetables and fruits every day, eating whole grains, eating healthy fats, and exercising for 30 minutes. The unhealthy habits are use of added sugar, snacking on anything other than fruits and vegetables, eating large amounts of non-vegetarian or milk products, eating out without following the diet, and watching television while eating. The next phase is all about keeping these habits for life, improving on them and increasing physical activity.

Not just another diet

Although it is quite popular, this diet is not like other run-of-the-mill diets. It won't keep you hooked for some time and eventually bore you or worse, not seem to have any effect. This diet has been carefully designed by experts from the Mayo Clinic. It is a result of judicious and relentless observation and research on the data of its patients over the years. The research focused on real people with weight issues, and observed what worked for them and what did not; the care and effort that have gone into formulating this diet is what gives it such reliability.

Not for everyone

This diet seems to be a one-stop solution for every Tom, Dick and Harry. But the truth is far from this assumption. Of course, if you are simply looking to lose weight while eating substantially or simply adopting a healthy lifestyle, you can go for it. But the myth that everyone should follow it is a cliché born out of lack of awareness. This diet focuses on low-calorie foods and very little amounts of meat, milk and dairy products. So it is not suitable for body-building professionals, athletes, pregnant women, and people with special medical conditions, and it might actually do them more harm than good. Also, it is quite tough to follow for hard-core non-vegetarians. This is because it concentrates more on veggies and fruits and wants you to have less of meat and dairy products. So, before you start this diet, discuss it with your doctor to confirm if it meets your specific criteria.

Not for instant weight loss

Although the first two-week phase (Lose it!) will most probably let you lose about 2 to 5 kg of weight, the subsequent weight loss is gradual. As it is a 'way of life' diet plan, you can expect to lose as little as 1 kg of body weight per month after the first phase, depending on your choices. Obviously, this is not meant for rapid results and is more suited for those who can persevere.

In fact, the initial weight loss that seems to be quite rewarding can be achieved by following most diet plans. This because when one first starts a diet, the initial weight loss is brought about by the breakdown of stored glucose in one's body. This breakdown is initiated when lesser calories are introduced suddenly along with increase in demand of calories (in the form of exercise). Obviously, this feature is present in every diet plan. The weight loss after that happens due to breakdown of stored fat in the body, which is tougher to achieve.

Not just a diet

Unlike other common diets, the Mayo Clinic diet is much more than just a way to watch what you are eating. As already mentioned, physical exercise is an integral part of this diet. In fact, it might not work at all if you don't include the exercising part and follow it regularly. But if followed properly, it can benefit you way beyond weight loss. It will improve your overall metabolism and digestion. It is also good for the heart and blood flow. Also, exercising regularly will improve your stamina and flexibility.

But there are some down sides as well. It will not be good for people with a weak skeletal or dental system. In particular, people with arthritis and women with osteoporosis and similar conditions should add more fats and proteins.

The above mentioned points likely contradicts many of the myths and rumors going around about the Mayo Clinic Diet. So based on these facts, you can plan your own version of the Mayo Clinic Diet as it is quite flexible. The Mayo Clinic has a special cookbook specifically for this diet, but it not all-inclusive. In fact, you can decide what recipes fits the bill and what does not by looking at the ingredients and calories. You can even improvise and modify your recipes to make them adhere to this diet.

Now, let us look at some recipes recommended by Mayo Clinic itself. Read on to learn and try these simple and delicious recipes to give you a kick-start to your diet plan.

RECIPES

Breakfast
One serving of fruit yogurt parfait

Ingredients
To prepare this, you will need:
Low-fat yogurt (plain or flavored)
Assorted fresh fruits (apple, banana, berries, etc.)
Low-fat granola.

Preparation
- Put a half cup of yogurt in a bowl or dish.
- Top it with a layer of assorted fruits.
- Top this with a layer of granola.
- Finally add some more yogurt and stir thoroughly.

Your yummy, low-calorie breakfast is ready.

Lunch
One serving of pasta and tuna salad and one orange.

Ingredients

To prepare the salad, you will need:

- 1 can tuna (water packed and drained)
- 4 cups of cooked shell pasta
- 2 cups of fresh chopped veggies (carrots, zucchini, iceberg lettuce, onions, peas, etc.)
- 4 tablespoons of a low-calorie salad dressing.

Preparation

- Put all the ingredients except the salad dressing in a large bowl and toss thoroughly.
- Add the dressing and mix well.

Dinner

For dinner, you can have **three slices of a 12-inch tomato basil pizza and a green salad.**

The salad can be prepared by mixing together assorted vegetables like red onions, cucumbers, and lettuce.

Ingredients

- 1 cup of wheat flour (whole grain)
- 1 cup of all-purpose flour
- ½ teaspoon each of salt and sugar
- 1 teaspoon each of yeast and olive oil

- 2 cups of crushed tomatoes (preferably fresh)
- 2/3 teaspoon each of dried basil and powdered black pepper
- ½ teaspoon of garlic powder
- some warm water
- 1 cup of reduced-fat cheese.

Preparation
- Preheat your oven to 375F.
- Mix the wheat flour, all-purpose flour, yeast, salt and sugar in a big bowl along with oil and water to prepare dough.
- Knead it thoroughly and add more flour or water gradually to achieve a non-sticky consistency.
- In a separate container, mix together the tomatoes and basil to prepare a paste.
- Add black pepper and garlic powder to the paste and mix well.
- Coat a pizza pan with cooking spray and roll out the dough onto it.
- Press the dough evenly and cover it with a layer of the tomato paste.
- Add a layer of grated cheese.
- Bake in the pre-heated oven for about 15 minutes until the dough gets brown.

So, with these and many such yummy and healthy recipes, you can embark upon a journey of a healthy lifestyle. All you have to do is update your grocery list, modify your recipes, redefine your servings and not compromise on your hunger. Happy (Mayo Clinic) dieting!

Chapter 13

Secrets about the TLC Diet

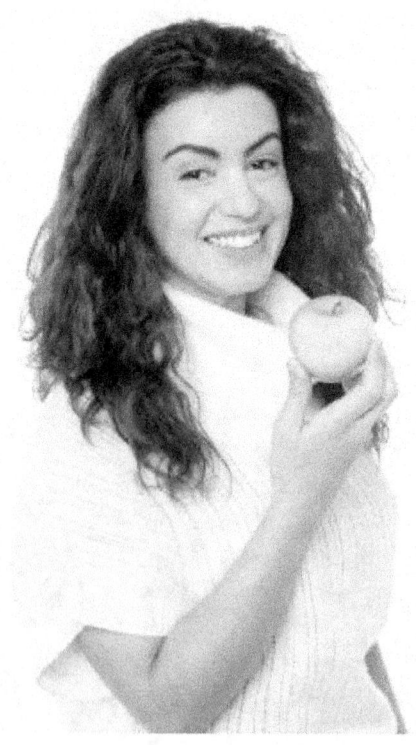

"Your body is a temple", said a great man. The Therapeutic Lifestyle Change Diet has been around since early 2004. Incepted by the US National Heart, Lung and Blood Institute, this diet helps to lower the risks of heart disease. While the aim of the diet isn't exactly to slim you down to size zero, it helps keep your diet and body weight in check.

With thousands of followers, this diet has been topping the charts of various wellness websites. To top it off, this diet ensures that one can change their life completely around, just by adopting the concept of careful eating.

#1.Claims of the diet:

The human body works on an intricate balance. This diet seeks to help people maintain an ideal balance between the array of things that they eat.

This diet targets more than just losing weight and cutting down fatty food. It is more holistic in its approach. The main causes of death in the US are heart attacks and high cholesterol levels. Even teenagers are becoming prone to heart attacks, thanks to diabetes and obesity.

All this can be traced to one main cause: unhealthy lifestyles.

The TLC diet is practiced in three stages:

Stage 1: The Diet
Stage 2: Physical Activities
Stage 3: Management of Weight

Through these three stages, the diet aims to lower the intake of LDL cholesterol, and hence, lower the risk of heart disease. (LDL cholesterol stands for low density lipoprotein. Commonly called the "bad cholesterol," LDL cholesterol gets deposited in parts of your body, causes clogging of arteries, and cannot be eliminated from the body easily.)

"How does cholesterol affect my heart?" you might ask.
Cholesterol is an oil-like substance that is found in all the cells of our body. They are carried in packages of protein and lipids to essential organs for secretion of certain fluids.

It flows in your bloodstream and it does not mix with the blood cells, like oil and water. When there is excess cholesterol in your body, it accumulates and attaches itself to the walls of arteries. This results in the narrowing of arteries, which prevents blood flow. Sometimes, when the walls of the artery are clogged up, a blood clot will form. This momentarily stops the flow of blood to your heart and causes heart attacks.

The TLC diet prescribes the optimum cholesterol intake as 200 mg/dL daily, and its various diet plans seek to help followers keep cholesterol levels under check.

The diet also calls for reducing the intake of saturated fats, which are found mostly in poultry and dairy products. There is a dire need to reduce the intake of these fats, as they are solid and cannot be broken down by the body easily. Added to this, foods with high saturated fats also have high cholesterol content.

The diet ranges in intensity, in the sense that it is does not have a set time-frame. In the first few weeks of adopting the diet, you have to work with your doctor and adopt a dietary plan. Then, you aim to integrate physical exercises so that you can maintain your health and burn excess fat.

By following the recommended plan, there is said to be a reduction of cholesterol by 8-10% in six weeks.

#2. Promotes general awareness about what you eat:

The one major benefit of undergoing this diet is that you become aware of what you eat. To keep fats and cholesterol under check, you have to eat carefully.

The manual does not list the cholesterol and trans-fat content of every single food item out there. So, the next time you go grocery shopping, you'll have to look at the nutrition label of the item that you are going to buy. This way, you learn to calculate the percentage of unsaturated fats in the food you eat and learn how to take it in moderation. Further, you are able to compare the products of many brands and pick the healthiest option.

The NHLBI gives a comprehensive image of how one is to go about reading food labels.

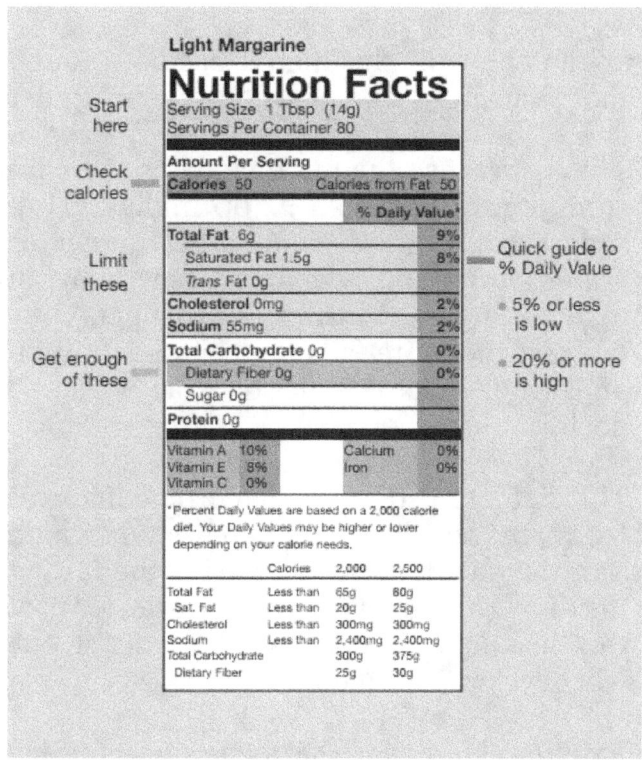

Light Margarine

Nutrition Facts

Serving Size 1 Tbsp (14g)
Servings Per Container 80

Amount Per Serving

Calories 50   Calories from Fat 50

% Daily Value*

Total Fat 6g	9%
Saturated Fat 1.5g	8%
Trans Fat 0g	
Cholesterol 0mg	2%
Sodium 55mg	2%
Total Carbohydrate 0g	0%
Dietary Fiber 0g	0%
Sugar 0g	
Protein 0g	

Vitamin A 10%	Calcium 0%
Vitamin E 8%	Iron 0%
Vitamin C 0%	

*Percent Daily Values are based on a 2,000 calorie diet. Your Daily Values may be higher or lower depending on your calorie needs.

	Calories	2,000	2,500
Total Fat	Less than	65g	80g
Sat. Fat	Less than	20g	25g
Cholesterol	Less than	300mg	300mg
Sodium	Less than	2,400mg	2,400mg
Total Carbohydrate		300g	375g
Dietary Fiber		25g	30g

Start here

Check calories

Limit these

Get enough of these

Quick guide to % Daily Value

• 5% or less is low

• 20% or more is high

#3. Comprehensive in nature:

The TLC diet isn't tailored to be followed for just a month or two. The diet mandates a change in one's lifestyle itself.

All this comes with enormous benefits such as weight loss, increase in stamina and decrease in cholesterol.
Although weight loss isn't the low-fat nature of this help in reducing weight.

http://www.nhl bi.nih.gov/healt

161

While following this diet, it has been found that not only is cholesterol kept under check, but sodium levels are also curbed. This is because the diet mandates the consumption of less than 2,300 milligrams of sodium daily. The focus is on eating whole grains, fruits and vegetables. This helps in maintaining a healthy and functioning body. It therefore falls under the definition of a "whole-hearted" diet plan, according to doctors.

The diet has also helped in curbing diabetes for many people. A US-based study found that this diet helped in lowering the fasting insulin levels in participants. The level of this insulin is important to predict if one will develop Type 2 diabetes.

Experts claim that the focus on shunning the wrong kinds of food, while emphasizing the right ones, is what makes this diet a success.

The NHLBI lists physical activities along with the extent of vigor and calories burnt. Based on the individual's existing health conditions, one can determine their workout regimen.

Burned in Common Activities

http://www.nhl bi.nih.gov/healt

Activity	
Walking (leisurely), 2 miles per hour	85
Walking (brisk), 4 miles per hour	170
Gardening	135
Raking leaves	145
Dancing	190
Bicycling (leisurely), 10 miles per hour	205
Swimming laps, medium level	240
Jogging, 5 miles per hour	275

*For a healthy 150-pound person. A lighter person burns fewer calories; a heavier person burns more.

Each of these activities burns approximately 150 calories:

Example of Moderate Amounts of Physical Activity

Common Chores	Sports Activities	Less Vigorous, More Time
Washing and waxing a car for 45–60 minutes	Playing volleyball for 45–60 minutes	↑
Washing windows or floors for 45–60 minutes	Playing touch football for 45 minutes	
Gardening for 30–45 minutes	Walking 1½ miles in 35 minutes (20 minutes/mile)	
Wheeling self in for wheelchair 30–40 minutes	Basketball (shooting baskets) for 30 minutes	
Pushing a stroller 1½ miles in 30 minutes	Bicycling 5 miles in 30 minutes	
Raking leaves for 30 minutes	Dancing fast (social) for 30 minutes	
Shoveling snow for 15 minutes	Walking 2 miles in 30 minutes (15 minutes/mile)	
Stair walking for 15 minutes	Water aerobics for 30 minutes	
	Swimming laps for 20 minutes	
	Basketball (playing game) for 15–20 minutes	
	Bicycling 4 miles in 15 minutes	
	Jumping rope for 15 minutes	
	Running 1½ miles in 15 minutes (10 minutes/mile)	More Vigorous, Less Time ↓

#4. What goes where?

Diets are designed with the concept of sacrifice in mind. If you want to gain something, you have to lose something else. The TLC diet ensures that you don't lose too much.

With such easy replacements, you won't regret going on this diet!

1. Replace beef and duck with the breast meats of chicken and turkey. Beef is high in saturated fats, which is the main cause of heart disease.

2. Fish has lower content of saturated fats than most kinds of meat. Shrimp is another variant that you can enjoy from time to time. While on this diet, you are to eat less than 200 mg of cholesterol daily. Three ounces of boiled shrimp is said to have 167 mg of cholesterol, so you're safe.

3. Switch from egg yolks to egg whites. The latter has no cholesterol, while yolks have around 213 mg per yolk. Ensure that you use egg whites for baking as well. Two egg whites make for a whole egg!

4. In the case of dairy products, one has to be extra careful. Make sure you buy fat-free milk and skim cheese, as they contain less fat. You might want to consider buying low-fat yogurt. Replacing your cheesy dips with salsa is also a good tip.

5. According to this diet, you should load yourself with fruits and vegetables. Following the dietary plan, have 3 to 5 servings of these every day. Replace your greasy snacks with assorted veggies dressed with lemon juice, herbs and spices.

#5. How does it work?

According to NHLBI, the TLC diet starts off by determining a goal for your daily calorie intake, which is 2,500 for men and 1,800 for women if your concern is just to reduce cholesterol. If weight loss is also desired, women should aim for 1,200 calories a day, and men for 1,600 calories a day.

According to the diet, the total saturated fat should amount to less than 7% of calories each day. You should consume less than 200 milligrams of saturated fat daily. The result after six weeks should be a reduction in cholesterol by 8-10%.

Through TLC, you combine various kinds of physical exercise. At the same time, you follow a balanced diet.

Although NHLBI gives an overview of saturated fat levels, the diet is highly individual-centric. Therefore, how you meet the guidelines is entirely up to you.

The diet combines this healthy intake with physical exercise, so that you can keep calories in check. Added to this, conditions like blood pressure, obesity and hypertension are all effectively prevented.

RECIPES

Breakfast
Oatmeal with bananas and cranberries
Cooking Time: 5 minutes

Ingredients
- 1 cup, Regular or fast-cooking oatmeal
- 2 cups, Low-fat or non-fat milk
- 1 cup, Cranberries, dried
- 1 Banana
- 1 tbsp honey

Preparation
Stove or Microwave
- Take a microwavable dish or a pot, and pour the oatmeal in.
- Next, pour the milk over the oatmeal. Remember, the ratio of milk to oatmeal should be 2:1.
- Then, add in the cranberries.
- Following this, place the dish over a stove or in a microwave for 2-3 minutes. Remember to keep a close watch on it as you do not want the milk to over flow!
- Once it is done, you can slice the bananas and add it to the bowl. An alternative would be to mash half the banana into the oatmeal mixture.

- Pour over the honey, mix, and enjoy.

Lunch
Bean and pea salad

Cooking time: 15-17 minutes

Ingredients
- 1 ½ cups, any kind of pea or bean
- 5 small-sized mushrooms, diced
- 1-2 medium sized leeks, sliced
- 1 medium-sized onion, sliced
- 3 cloves of garlic, chopped finely
- Seasoning-Pepper and sea salt

Preparation
- Sautee the mushrooms for a few minutes until they are completely cooked. When they are cooked, the mushrooms will be soft.
- Then, pour in your sliced onions, leeks and the chopped garlic.
- Add the required amount of salt and pepper, and stir for a few minutes. Remove from heat, once done.
- In the meanwhile, boil the peas or beans that you are going to add to your vegetables.
- Once boiled, drain excess water and pour into the serving dish.
- Season the beans with desired amount of salt.

- Add the vegetables to the beans, mix thoroughly.
- Then, serve.

Note: This dish goes great with boiled or steamed turkey breasts, seasoned lightly.

Dinner
Stew with lentils, tomatoes and on-ions

Cooking Time: Approximately 1 hour and 15 minutes

Ingredients
- 2-3 carrots, diced or sliced
- 1 cup tomatoes, crushed
- 1/2 tsp sage
- 3 Teaspoons, olive oil
- 3/4th cup washed lentils
- 3 cups water
- 1 cup of peas-Optional
- 3/4th tsp ground ginger
- 2-3 medium sized onions
- 3/4th tsp cumin
- 3/4th tsp salt
- 2 cups diced mushrooms

Preparation
- Take two teaspoons of oil and heat it over medium flame. Slowly add the

sliced garlic and diced carrots and cook for five minutes, until soft.

- Pour in crushed tomatoes, lentils, salt, cumin, mushrooms, ginger and sage. Add the cups of water and turn upto a high flame.
- Once boiled, turn to simmer, and cook for 30-35 minutes, until the lentils are cooked.
- In a pan, heat 1 spoon of oil, and add onions and sugar. Cook for five minutes, while stirring constantly. At the end of this time, the onions will be dark gold in color.
- Optional: Pour in the peas and add it to the stew. Cook for 2-3 minutes.
- Garnish the stew with the golden onions, and then serve.

Chapter 14

Secrets about the Volumetrics Diet

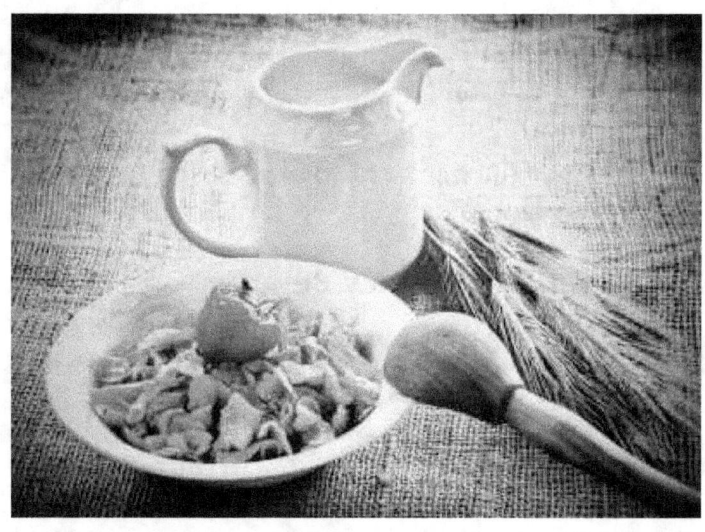

The Volumetrics diet is one of the top-ranking diets. Barbara Rolls came up with this diet in 2000. The Volumetric diet helps in losing a pound or two per week. It is very different from crash diets. This diet does not cut down or restrict high-fat foods.

Instead, it focuses on the amount consumed. It allows you to eat more low-calorie foods and limited high-calorie foods. So when you eat lots of low-calorie foods, you tend to think you're full. This diet suggests that you take in water-rich fruits and vegetables, soups, and salads, since water has zero calories and gets easily absorbed.

This might make you hungry again, but your body gets fooled into thinking you are eating a lot, while you're cutting down on calories. This diet might take a while to adjust to, particularly for those who overeat. Professional help is a better choice.

Claims & Primary Benefits

The Volumetrics diet is a diet in which a person consumes more food with low energy density. This way, he feels fuller and more satisfied, unlike crash diets, and so this helps a person to lose weight by eating more.

The Volumetrics diet focuses on creating a healthier lifestyle rather than abruptly bringing down the weight, so weight loss occurs gradually; one can be expected to lose a pound or two per week. Moreover, as opposed to restricted diets or crash diets that bring people back to their unhealthy eating habits after they fail to follow it, with the Volumetrics diet, no food is strictly banned; only the amount is restricted.

Additional Benefits

Since this diet reduces the intake of salt and saturated fats, it maintains the cholesterol and blood pressure level and prevents heart-related problems. It does not have any side effects, and it is suitable for all ages. Following this diet also reduces the risk of type 2 diabetes.

How Does the Diet Work?

The main highlight of this diet is that it encourages the intake of food with lower energy density. Those that are less energy dense are foods that have lesser number of calories for a specific weight. This diet recommends water-rich foods such as fruits and vegetables, broth-based soups, lean meat and whole grains, which make you feel fuller even though they are lighter in calories.

But foods that are high in calories such as fried foods and candy will not satisfy your hunger, though the calorie intake keeps increasing. So this diet encourages eating large amounts of low-calorie foods rather than eating a small amount of high-calorie food.

The cost incurred during the Volumetrics diet is less, since it mostly suggests home-made food. This diet will reduce hunger, depression and tiredness.

Classification of food based on energy density:

Food can be classified based on their energy densities into four categories:

Category 1: Fruits and Vegetables. They can be consumed in any amount.
Category 2: Whole grains, low-fat dairy, legumes and lean proteins like poultry, tofu and seafood. They can be consumed in reasonable quantities.
Category 3: Breads, desserts, cheese, fat-free snacks and meat. They can be consumed in small quantities.
Category 4: Fried foods, cookies, nuts, high-calorie desserts and fats. They have to be consumed in minimal quantities.
Foods under category 1 and category 2 are encouraged. Category 3 foods can be con-

sumed once in a while. It is best that foods under category 4 are avoided.

The diet should be accompanied by 30-60 minutes of daily exercise. Maintaining a journal to record your eating habits and exercise routine will help you stay on track and watch your progress.

Facts & Figures

You can lose 1-2 pounds per week on the Volumetrics diet
According to the 2010 Dietary Guidelines for Americans, 20-35% of the daily calories should be from fat, and 45-65% of the calories should be from carbohydrates.

Acceptable intake level of sodium is 2,300 milligrams, and if you have heart ailments or if you are over the age of 50, the level of recommended sodium intake is reduced to 1,500 milligrams. To reduce the salt intake, processed foods should be avoided.

Around 22 to 34 grams of fiber should be consumed per day. Fruits, vegetables, whole grains and beans are major sources of fiber.

It is recommended that you consume 4,700 milligrams of potassium per day, but it is not easy to meet this requirement. Although bananas are rich in potassium, it would take 11 bananas to meet that demand. Though the recommended amount of potassium may not be consumed, eating a lot of fruits and vegetables will certainly increase the potassium intake.

It is necessary to consume 1,000-1,300 milligrams of calcium per day. Low-fat dairy products should be introduced in your diet to meet the calcium requirement.
Adults need 2.4 micrograms of Vitamin B12. It is essential for proper cell metabolism. Yogurt, salmon, trout and fortified cereals are good sources of Vitamin B12.

Those who do not get adequate sunlight to receive the recommended 15 milligrams of Vitamin D need to include low-fat dairy, fortified cereals or supplements in their diet to lower the risk of bone fractures.

The Volumetrics diet satisfies all these guidelines. It gives you all the essential nutrients, even as you lose weight.

Additional Tips

Various plans are available. A 1,600-calorie plan would have a 400-calorie breakfast, 500-calorie lunch, 200-calorie snack and a 500-calorie dinner. Very few calories per day will strip you of the nutrients required to keep your body going, so it is necessary for every individual to consume a minimum of 1,200 calories per day. Calculate the amount of calories you can consume per day based on your height, weight and activity level. If you cut down your calorie intake by 500 calories per day, you will lose a pound or two per week. This diet gives you a menu from which you can make choices for breakfast, lunch, snacks and dinner each day.

For example, on a particular day, your meal plan may be:

Breakfast: Cereal with fruit and skimmed milk
Lunch: Vegetable soup, vegetable sandwich, lean roast beef and an apple
Snack: Any fruit with yogurt
Dinner: Salad, pasta primavera, pumpkin custard

RECIPES

Here are some simple easy-to-do recipes for breakfast, lunch, snack and dinner.

Breakfast
Carrot Soup

Ingredients
- 1 potato
- Red lentils
- Stock cubes
- A few carrots
- Chilli powder
- 1 garlic clove
- Cabbage
- Broccoli
- Salt
- Pepper

Preparation

Chop the potatoes into cubes and fry them in a pan. After a few minutes, add boiling water to the pan and crumble in stock cubes. Add the lentils. Mix in the chili powder. Grate the carrots to save cooking time and add them to the pan. Next chop the garlic clove and add the cabbage after cutting it.

Lastly, add the broccoli. Allow mixture to boil for 15-20 minutes. Your soup is ready to be served.

Lunch
Sandwich

Ingredients
- 3 slices of brown bread

- 1 egg

- 1 tomato, thinly sliced

- 1 onion, thinly sliced

- 4 cheese slices (cheddar or mozzarella)

- 1 tablespoon mayonnaise

- Ketchup

- Lemon juice

- Black pepper

Preparation

Toast the bread slices until golden but not too crispy. Fry the egg and sprinkle salt and black pepper on it. Apply the mayonnaise over two bread slices, on one side. Assemble the sandwich in this manner: two cheese slices on the bread, followed by a layer of thinly sliced tomato and thinly sliced onion. Top this with the bread slice that does not have mayonnaise on it, and after that place the fried egg, followed by a layer of thinly sliced onion and again a layer of thinly sliced tomato. Place two cheese slices over this and complete the sandwich with the last slice of bread (with tomato ketchup). Grill the sandwich if you like, and raise the temperature to make sure the cheese melts!

Snack
Smoothie

Ingredients
- 2 bananas
- 2 handfuls of baby spinach
- 2 apples
- 1 cup of yogurt
- 6 strawberries
- 1/2 orange

Preparation

In a blender, place two handfuls of baby spinach, 2 apples, 2 bananas, 1 cup of yogurt, 6 strawberries, and a ½ of an orange. Blend to your desired consistency, and your yummy smoothie is ready. Smoothies make you feel fuller and give you a lot of energy.

Dinner
Fruit-Veggie Salad

- 2 tomatoes, chopped

- 1 teaspoonof ginger garlic paste

- 1 cup of onion, chopped

- 1 cup of cucumber, grated

- 2 cups of yogurt

- 1 cup of pomegranate

- 1 cup of coriander leaves

- Salt

- 1 cup of carrot, grated

- 2 chillies, chopped

Preparation

First, mix the chopped tomatoes, chopped chillies, grated cucumber, grated carrots and onion in a bowl. Add salt, then yoghurt and ginger garlic paste to the mixture and mix well. Add the pomegranate and mix again. Finally top with coriander leaves and serve.

Never knew dieting could be this easy? Now you know! Follow this diet and watch those pounds shed away effortlessly. Good luck!

Chapter 15

Secrets about the Paleo Diet

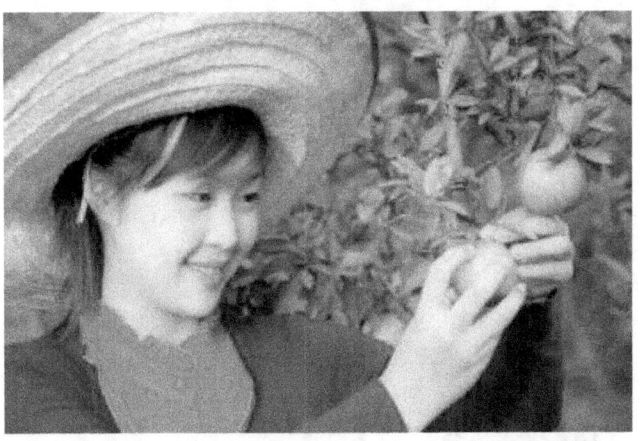

The evolution of man is fascinating. Our forefathers were hunters and gatherers, and were said to be lithe, strong, adaptive, and most of all, extremely healthy. Meat, vegetables and fruits made up the staple diet of a Paleolithic man.

Scientists, dietitians and fitness experts have formulated hundreds of diets to help us stay fit. Many diets out there solely focus on reducing weight by limiting the portion of food you eat.

In contrast, this diet was conceptualized by Loren Cordain and his team because they believed that human beings can achieve optimum health by eating what they are genetically fit to consume. What Paleo experts have deduced is that if we eat the way our forefathers ate, we can be as agile and strong as them. Their belief is that the human body is still not completely evolved to eat all kinds of food.

The diet is relatively low-key, but the benefits are plenty.
You might be thinking: "What? Why should I eat like a caveman? No way." Here are a few secrets that will change your mind.

#1. Premise:

The diet stands on just one motto, or rather, belief. It is that the best diet is one that we are genetically tailored to. The Paleo diet stresses eating vegetables, fruits and meat while shunning processed food.

Studies state that our bodies are not yet completely evolved and therefore unable to digest whole grains and processed foods. Experts have pointed out that health deterioration was due to the agricultural revolution.

While Paleolithic men were hunters and gatherers, modern men moved on to become farmers. During this period, they began cultivating wheat, paddy, rice and other food grains. Needless to say, they began to consume them as well. They expanded their palate, which their genetics were not adapted to.

And this tradition has continued until today. Our bodies are susceptible to multiple diseases, and obesity is the king of them all.

How can they say that agriculture ruined it all? Paleo experts state that most grains are glutinous and have lectins.

Grains have their own body system. The structures of grains have progressed in a way such that they aren't eaten. Lectin is a toxin that protects grains from being eaten. Further, they prevent our intestinal tract from repairing itself. Gluten, on the other hand, is a protein that the human body isn't fully evolved to digest. Gluten allergy is still prevalent. In addition, it causes an array of diseases like osteoporosis and heart disease.

In a nutshell, the diet says NO processed food, NO artificial sugar and NO grains.

#2. How does it work?

Our bodies are designed in a magnificent manner.

We believe that while on a diet, we should reduce our carbohydrate intake. This diet, however, is based on one simple guideline: we should eat what our bodies were genetically adapted to eat. It stresses the fact that diets cannot just shun carbohydrates away. What they should focus on is the consumption of carbohydrates that can be broken down easily.

Even if our body has low levels of carbohydrates, it will function adequately, because our body simply burns stored fat to keep itself functioning smoothly.

Thus, less glucose equals more fat being burned. Easy, right?

Well, think again. Since we are so used to consuming grains, cereals and pastries, we are stuck with excess carbohydrates. Simply put, our bodies are being piled up with carbs, and we aren't able to burn it all away.

When our bodies cannot burn it away, it gets deposited as fat. The more this happens, the more overweight we tend to become.

Following this diet would mean you condemn all sources of carbohydrates that are processed in any way. Thus, the sources from which you derive carbohydrates should be au natural - fruits, vegetables and meat. The diet also mandates a good source of protein. Try combining eggs, pork, fish and chicken with each meal. This way, you have a balanced diet.

Another important Paleo guideline is to stay away from most forms of dairy products. Historically, no animal drinks milk beyond the stage of infancy. Paleolithic men didn't carry around cows for milk. The Paleo diet insists that our bodies aren't fully evolved to digest milk. The diet states that this is why there is lactose intolerance.

This has two-fold benefits. One, you get the required level of energy by eating these foods. Secondly, when it comes to these sources, there isn't room for over-eating.

Even while eating meat, ensure that you don't soak the dish in oil.

What Paleo dietitians tell us to do is to eat until we're full. And when meat is combined with vegetables, we won't binge more than necessary.

#3. What should you eat?

By now you might be mind-boggled. In fact, the entire idea of the diet might seem baffling. After all, how can you just live on unprocessed meat? The diet also states that you shouldn't consume any artificial forms of sugar. How do you eat freely then?

But you needn't limit yourself; there are so many things to eat while staying healthy.

-        In the case of meat, make sure the poultry is grass-fed. Grain-fed animals have the same problems that humans do. The grains that are fed to them will be transferred to you indirectly.

-        You can eat eggs, but the dietary guidelines ask you to look for eggs enriched with Omega-3.

-        You are advised to eat all kinds of fruit while on this diet. They will be your

188

primary source of sugar. If your goal is to lose weight, you should watch fruit intake as they are higher in calories.

-        Eat a lot of vegetables; pile them up on your plate. Make sure that they aren't deep-fried. Also, add plenty of yams and sweet potatoes to your meals. These kinds of vegetables are high in carbohydrates. The caloric intake is also higher, and this way, you will still sustain the same energy level throughout the day.

-        Natural oils such as coconut oil and olive oil can be used for cooking. Again, these should be used in moderation.

-        Since toxins can be found in canned and farmed fish, pick wild fish for meals.

-        The Paleo diet encourages you to eat nuts, as they are relatively healthier than many other snack options. However, these should be consumed in moderation, as they are processed to some extent.

-        Replace cow's milk with almond milk.

#4. How will I stay fit if I eat this way?

Well, this is a valid question. All this information might still not be convincing.

Eating chips is a habit amongst all of us. Just think about the number of packets you had to eat to become full. Maybe 3 or 4, right?

Now, let's paint another picture. An oven-roasted steak with boiled vegetables can fill you up with just one or two servings. Even in cases of extreme hunger, you can eat a few servings and it won't hurt your health.

While studying the benefits of this diet, doctors saw that eating the latter kept you full for hours. On the other hand, the chips will immediately make you feel hungry in another forty minutes. It was noticed that followers of this diet were able to reduce weight in just a few weeks.

#5. Some tips to follow:

Give the diet thirty days: When you shift over to a diet like this, the transition might not be that easy. The sudden drop in carbohydrate intake might make you a bit sluggish. Keep eating the grass-fed meat and stack up vegetables on your plate. In fact, try taking a picture of yourself at the beginning of the month. Don't give up, try the diet and snap a picture at the end of the month. Compare the two pictures and see for yourself how the diet has impacted your body.

Weight loss isn't the first item on the list: We have been eating unhealthily for many years now. This diet will help you increase your metabolism, but the point isn't to shed pounds. This is a way to change your lifestyle for good. You will be stronger and more energetic. That's the priority right now!

Experiment and experiment more: You might feel like your freedom is being held captive, but don't give in. Have an open mind and keep trying out new recipes. Experiment with different fruits and vegetables, and have fun eating.

RECIPES

Breakfast
Scrambled eggs with Kale

Ingredients
- 4, Omega-3 eggs
- 4, Kale leaves (Large)
- A pinch of sea salt
- Olive or coconut oil

Preparation
- Take eggs and crack them open into a blender.
- Take the Kale leaves and drop into the same blender.
- Add salt, and then blend until the mixture is smooth.
- Heat oil in a pan over medium flame.
- Once the oil is hot, pour the mixture to the pan.
- Cook the eggs and scramble.
- Once it reaches your desired level of cooking, turn off the flame.
- Serve with steamed vegetables or meat.

Lunch
Currant and Spinach salad

Ingredients

- 5 cups, spinach
- One-fourth cup, currants
- 1 apple, sliced into thin strips
- 1 cup, broken walnuts
- 2 tbsp, olive oil
- 2 tbsp, balsamic vinegar

Preparation
- In a bowl, mix the spinach, currants and apple.
- Toast walnuts over low-flame for about 8 minutes.
- Dress the salad with olive oil and vinegar.
- Then, add the walnuts.
- Toss the salad thoroughly, and serve.

Dinner:
Zesty Chicken with Lime

Ingredients
- 1.5 kilograms chicken pieces, with bones
- 12 slices of halved lime
- 1 tbsp, paprika
- 2 tbsp, coconut sugar or alternative
- 1 tbsp, garlic powder
- 1 tsp, allspice
- 1 tbsp, black pepper, grounded
- Half tsp, ground Celtic sea salt

Preparation

- Take chicken pieces, place with limes in a bowl.
- In another container, mix paprika, salt, pepper, coconut sugar, allspice, garlic powder and mix.
- Pour the spice mix over the chicken uniformly and mix.
- Cook the chicken on a barbecue grill for 30-40 minutes, giving 15-20 minutes for each side. The side which is cooking should be face-down.
- Serve it hot.

Conclusion

I hope this book was worth your time. Please forgive me if there were any errors as this is my first book.

Feel free to leave a review. I pretty excited to hear your feedback.

I am writing the 2nd part of the series. It's almost complete. I should be able to publish it within a month.

<u>Image Credits</u> via freedigitalphotos.net

Photos by stockimages, marin, Apolonia, Sura Nualpradid, zirconicusso, imageryma-jestic, Serge Bertasius Photography, Apolonia, Serge Bertasius Photography, and Grant Cochrane